MEDICINE AND CHRISTIAN MORALITY

MEDICINE AND CHRISTIAN MORALITY

THOMAS J. O'DONNELL, S.J.

ALBA · HOUSE NEW · YORK

SOCIETY OF ST. PAUL, 2187 VICTORY BLVD., STATEN ISLAND, NEW YORK 10314

Library of Congress Cataloging in Publication Data
O'Donnell, Thomas Joseph, 1918-
    Medicine and Christian Morality.
    Includes index.
    1. Medical ethics.   2.   Christian ethics-
Catholic authors.   I. Title.   [DNLM: 1. Catholicism.
2. Ethics, Medical. 3. Religion and medicine.
W50 026m]
R724.028   174'.2   75-41471
ISBN 0-8189-0323-6

Nihil Obstat:
+ George E. Lynch
Censor Librorum

Imprimatur:
✠ F. Joseph Gossman
Bishop of Raleigh, N.C.
December 8, 1975

*The Nihil Obstat and Imprimatur
are a declaration that a book or pamphlet is considered
to be free from doctrinal or moral error. It is not implied that
those who have granted the Nihil Obstat and Imprimatur agree
with the contents, opinions or statements expressed.*

Designed, printed and bound in the United States of
America by the Fathers and Brothers of the Society of St. Paul,
2187 Victory Boulevard, Staten Island, New York, 10314,
as part of their communications apostolate.

1 2 3 4 5 6 7 8 9 (Current Printing: first digit).

INTRODUCTION

The recasting of a Medical-Moral text that was first taking shape almost twenty-five years ago may seem analogous to something like the Pick's and Alzheimer's syndrome reflected in an ethico-moral context. One might wonder if the dramatic and widely publicized ethical and theological speculations of the last decade have left all previous thinking in a state of premature senility, apathy, immobility, and perhaps even well deserved mutism, or if the attempt to renew the traditional ethico-moral context is doomed to a certain pointless hyperactivity and restlessness.

It must be frankly admitted that bringing forth this text, even though it is conceived in the context of Catholic Moral Theology, presents special problems even on its home grounds. This is because it is a didactic work presented in the atmosphere of the renewed kerygmatic consciousness of the contemporary Church.

Kerygma and *didache* might best be identified respectively as *preaching* and *teaching*. The kerygmatic proclamation of the "good news" of the Christian evangel is the presentation of the gospel in a way that man may be moved to believe—to accept and to adhere to the community of believers. In this concept, as Avery Dulles points out, the Church is not so much a school as a community of believers. Here there is an emphasis and style of approach that is somewhat different from the ecclesial *didache*. The didactic mission of the Church consists rather in the interpretation of the basic evangelical proclamation, seeking to logically explore and reasonably present the more detailed implications of the gospel in the daily life of contemporary man.

The Christian Revelation, of course, does not contain explicitly all the answers to life's questions—indeed, it does not even propose all the questions. There is no doubt that theologians have got into trouble at times by overscoping the content of revelation—by wrongly trying to identify, in the message, either implicit or explicit answers to questions that are not really treated there. This is fundamentally what happened in the Church's unfortunate and humiliating battles with Copernicus, Galileo and Darwin.

Yet there is an equal danger of under-scoping. There is no doubt that some of the manualists, in times past, confused and distorted the law of love by pushing it too deeply into Aristotelian categories. But this unfortunate overkill does not change the fact that the gospel teachings and the fundamental facts of human rights and obligations are not always practically evident in each emotion charged human situation. There are times when carefully reasoned analyses are required.

It is true that the most fundamental dimension of true human living lies in an openness to life—to the Father's love for us and our love for one another, but Augustine's *"Ama, et fac quod vis"* is not enough for most of us. In the ordinary life of the ordinary man there are just too many deceptive, apparent, immediate, pseudo-goods which distort our moral evaluations and limit our openness. Here the *didache* still has a vitally important purpose to serve, in delineating the objectively "morally good" and "morally bad." These pages are designed to help to serve that purpose.

Although this book began as a third revision of my original text: *Morals in Medicine* (Westminster, The Newman Press, 1956; Second, Revised and Enlarged Edition, 1959), I have given it a new title: *Medicine and Christian Morality*. I believe that this new title represents a more honest confrontation with our contemporary scene. Although new and contemporary questions are evaluated, it is not meant to be, primarily, an exploration of new theological frontiers. My purpose is simply to relate Catholic doctrine to the field of Medical Ethics, and to shed some light on the many areas of speculation within dimensions congruent with authentic Catholic teaching. For Catholics, this book is meant to be a guide. For non-Catholics it will hopefully be a source of significant information.

TABLE OF CONTENTS

MEDICINE AND CHRISTIAN MORALITY

CHAPTER ONE

THE BACKGROUND

The medical literature of the past decade has carried an increasing number of articles dealing with medical ethics. But exactly what is medical ethics? Or rather should the question be, "What *are* medical ethics?" Are we speaking of one thing, or of several things—and this suggests another and perhaps the most pregnant question of all: "Is there really an ethic which is medical?"

When Paul of Tarsus wrote a letter to his converts at Rome, parts of it read strangely like parts of the modern novel, which so often portrays contemporary decadence that a Harvard professor can wonder whether it is already too late "to strengthen the web of morality which enables society to perpetuate itself."[1]

It seems to me that if we say medical ethics *is* thus and so, we are implying a unity which we deem appropriate and would like to see verified; but which *de facto* does not exist. In our deontological pluralism, the only way that we can enuntiate any moral code that is acceptable to all, is in the most general terms of doing good and avoiding evil. Not far beyond that generality we run into the problem of divergent value-systems in human society—a divergence inherent in the diversity of meanings which men impose upon the operative words: good and evil, as well as variations of the relative importance of the many goods and evils within a particular value-system.

This is demonstrated by the existence, even within the restricted field of Medicine, of a number of different codes such as the American Medical Association Code, The World Health Organization Code, The American Hospital Association Code, as well as those other codes whose dimensions are more directly and deeply influenced by various theological convictions.

Of course there are those who would say that no theological consideration should enter the picture, but that is easier said than done. A strictly non-theological frame of reference must ultimately rest on a sort of atheism which leaves morality without any anchor. Ethics is not theology, but it cannot survive without some supporting theism. Even our American Bill of Rights rests on the theistic foundation of the Declaration of Independence. Perhaps the real questions are: first, where does ethics live? and now is there one Medical Ethic, or are there many Medical Ethics, or is there, properly speaking, any Medical Ethic?

Where ethics lives is at the heart of man, based on his most fundamental response to the meaning of life. His ethic is his concern for the moral goodness of what he does—that certain supra-sensible quality of any human choice whereby we measure it against a supra-sensible norm of good or bad.

"Good" and "bad," in an ethical context, are value words, and value implies desirability. A man desires what he recognizes as good, within his scale of values. The recognized good is the recognized value—and is the reason why the object or action is desired—and this immediately introduces the very personal dimension of what the individual conceives as valuable to himself, both in himself and consistent with all the desirable relationships to which he responds in human life. Even the law of genuine love rests on the apparent (and only apparent) contradiction that to selflessly seek the good of the beloved is the deepest self-fulfillment. That is the anatomy of an ethic.

But there is a difference between "Medical Ethics" as value judgments *arising only from* concepts exclusively proper to the practice of Medicine, and the broader ethical and moral convictions of individuals *as they relate to* the practice of Medicine.

Is there, then, one Medical Ethic, which is derived from and proper to Medicine itself? Howard Taylor seems to say that there is in a recent essay on "The Ethics of the Physician in Human Reproduction," in which he describes the sources of Medical Ethics as: "a few essential principles so clearly inherent in the doctor-patient relationship that they continue to recur in each new form of society."[2] Thus he seems to be referring to a sort of quintessence of strictly *Medical* Ethics, evident in the very nature and purpose of medical practice. Among the examples of such principles he mentions the priority of the patient's welfare. But then Dr. Taylor adds (and I believe most significantly and very much to our point), "(These) have always been interpreted in the light of our current theological and social values and . . . these are subject to constant change."

It is not difficult to see how social and theological divergencies can modify the principle of the priority of the patient's welfare. Consider the case of the reluctant pregnant mother, where one obstetrician considers himself to be treating the clinical welfare of only one patient, while another obstetrician sees himself as the guardian of two lives. The first might see abortion as something therapeutic and good, while the second would see it as destructive and bad, and hardly conducive to the welfare of the smaller patient.

This case points to a basic question: is there one Medical Ethic, or two Medical Ethics, or no *Medical* Ethics, properly so-called? I am inclined to think that the third option brings us closest to the truth.

The nature of any profession is the service of one's fellow man in an area of some sophisticated expertise—a service that is seen as essential to the good of the community. Thus I would be willing to admit that there is a professional ethic, but deriving from the nature of profession, rather than from the nature of medicine, and equally applicable to all of the professions. Such an ethic would deal with the modalities of client-centered services, freedom from economic venality, or personal aggrandizement as determining or limiting one's service to one's fellow man, a professional reticence regarding the confidentialities exposed in serving others, self-perpetuation of the profession, and the like. Such an ethic applies equally to the professions of law, medicine, ministry, education, and so forth. Nor does it seem to me that the practice of Medicine, as a profession, requires any specific professional ethic peculiar to itself. Rather there is a sort of fundamental ethic, or sub-ethic, arising from the nature of any profession and applicable to all professions equally.

In addition to this sub-ethic, fundamental to all the professions and peculiar to none, there is likewise a supra-ethic: that is, an ethical orientation of every thinking man that is derived from his understanding of the meaning of human life and human living, which consists of the moral values that he has built into his life. This ethic will bring certain specifications into the medical context, whether the individual is giving or receiving in the therapeutic process.

It is clear that there can be no universal codifications of these ethical and religious values in a pluralistic society. Such values, as realized in the therapeutic regimen, have been erroneously called "Jewish Medical Ethics," or "Catholic Medical Ethics," and so on. I say "erroneously" because there is no Catholic Medicine, or Jewish Medicine, or Jehovah's Witness Medicine.

That is why there is a striking accuracy in the official title of a document recently approved by the Bishops of the United States—called: *Ethical and Religious Directives for Catholic Health Facilities.* This is better than entitling the document: "Medical Ethics," because its directives are not derived precisely and exclusively from the art and science of Medicine. They are derived from broader philosophical and theological principles as applied to the practice of Medicine.

This is why a study of Medicine and Christian Morality must begin with some fundamental concepts of Christian Morality.

Fundamental Truths

The study of Ethics is an investigation into the goodness or evil of human actions in the light of natural reason. Moral Theology, on the other hand, investigates the morality of human actions against the background of man's supernatural life and destiny, and with the added assistance of divine revelation. The study of Canon Law is an investigation into the meaning and interpretation of the positive ecclesiastical law, which governs the external conduct of the baptized as members of the Catholic Church.

Each of these disciplines: Ethics, Moral Theology, and Canon Law, is concerned primarily with human conduct. The purpose of this book is to select some of the salient features of these three disciplines, as they relate to the therapeutic and research aspects of the art and science of Medicine.

For those who have not studied the related subjects which serve as a foundation for these considerations, some conclusions have been selected from basic studies which are mainly concerned with the nature of God and the nature of man, together with the broad impact of these considerations upon all human conduct. These can, in part, be summed up in the following excerpts from a previous statement of the Bishops of the United States:

How can man know what is his place in the divine plan, and what is God's Will in the moral decisions he is called upon to make? God has endowed man with intelligence. When rightly used and directed, the human intellect can discover certain fundamental spiritual truths and moral principles, which will give order and harmony to man's intellectual and moral life.

What are these truths which right reason can discover? First in importance is the existence of a personal God, all knowing and all powerful, the eternal Source from Whom all things derive their being. Next comes the spiritual and immortal nature of man's soul, its freedom, its responsibility, and the duty of rendering to God reverence, obedience, and all that is embraced under the name of religion.

From man's position as God's rational, free and responsible creature, destined for eternal life, spring the unique dignity of the human individual and his essential equality with his fellow men . . .

These are some of the basic elements of the natural law, a law based on human nature; a law which can be discovered by human intelligence and which governs man's relationship with God, with himself, and with the other creatures of God. The principles of the natural law, absolute, stable and unchangeable, are applicable to all the changing conditions and circumstances in which man constantly finds himself.

These religious and moral truths of the natural order can be known by human reason; but God, in His goodness, through Divine Revelation, has helped man to know better and to preserve the natural law. In the Old Testament this revelation was given to God's chosen people. Completed and perfected in the new, it has been communicated to mankind by Jesus Christ and His Apostles, and has been entrusted to the Church which Christ Himself established to teach all men . . .

Man must either acknowledge that a personal God exists, or he must deny His existence altogether. There is no middle course. Once he acknowledges that God exists, then the claims of God are co-extensive with all the activities of His creatures. To pretend that any part of life can be a private affair, is to violate the most basic claim which God has on man. Man is a creature. As a creature, he is subject to his Creator in all that he does. There is no time in his life when he is excused from obeying the moral law.[3]

To enucleate the proofs and demonstrations of these points does not fall within the subject matter of the moral aspects of medicine. In the following pages there will be found only selected and summary considerations of the general notions, which are most germane to the specific ethical questions subsequently treated. These will include the Church's image of herself in her nature, her teaching mission, and the media of that teaching, and the idea of God's law in the world of men. Moreover we will look briefly at the nature of law, in itself, in its relationship to the common good and to the individual. We will consider those diagnostic features which are called the determinants of morality, or those elements which enter into a moral choice, and by which its moral goodness or badness is determined and discerned. And finally in this chapter we will recall some of those psychosomatic modifications of the human personality, which sometimes and to some degree limit man's freedom to choose, and so likewise modify the responsibility of his choice.

For the believing Catholic, the Church is the sacrament of salvation. It is the Christ-willed and Christ-assisted continuation of His Galilean ministry and redemptive sacrifice, His love of mankind and His obedience to the eternal Father, continuing on through the centuries of human history.

The message and meaning of the Church is not confined to the Catholic—to the faithful who are the Church. As the Fathers of the Second Vatican Council made clear, the Church speaks to all who invoke the name of Christ, and to the whole human family, to the world of men; offering honest assistance to fostering the brotherhood of all mankind and, like its Founder (Jesus Christ), strives "to give witness to the truth, to rescue and not to sit in judgment, to serve and not to be served."[4]

It is the mission of the Church to bring to mankind the light enkindled in the gospel of the Lord Jesus, and as the same Council states, to put at mankind's disposal, "those saving resources which the Church herself, under the guidance of the Holy Spirit, receives from her Founder."[5]

The Media of the Church's Message

Everyone knows that the Catholic Church claims an authority, and indeed in some instances an infallibility, in teaching the revealed doctrine of Jesus Christ, and a prerogative of imparting the implications of that message to the modern world. It is unfortunate, however, that many have an erroneous and distorted idea of this concept. Although, as of this date, there is no teaching, proper and specific to the field of medical morality, which has been taught as infallible, a brief summary of the teaching of infallibility is important because of the many misunderstandings and distortions of this doctrine, that have always existed.

The doctrine was clearly defined at the First Vatican Council in the following classic passage:

We teach and define it to be a dogma divinely revealed that the Roman Pontiff, when he speaks *ex cathedra*, that is, when acting in his office as pastor and teacher of all Christians, by his supreme apostolic authority, he defines a doctrine concerning faith and morals to be held by the whole Church, through the divine assistance promised him in blessed Peter, he enjoys that infallibility with which the divine Redeemer willed His Church to be endowed in defining doctrine concerning faith and morals.[6]

And Vatican II reaffirmed the doctrine and made the role of the bishops explicit in the following passage:

This is the infallibility which the Roman Pontiff, the head of the college of Bishops, enjoys in virtue of his office, when as the supreme shepherd and teacher of all the faithful, who confirms his brethren in their faith (cf. Lk. 22:32), he proclaims by a definitive act some doctrine of faith or morals . . . The infallibility promised to the Church resides also in the body of bishops, when that body exercises supreme teaching authority with the successor of Peter.[7]

Thus it is clear that in Catholic doctrine this charism of infallibility, which the Church recognizes in both scripture and tradition, resides in the Roman Pontiff, and is exercised by him in what are properly called *ex cathedra* definitions, and is likewise shared by the college of Bishops, when explicitly in virtue of this charism, they are teaching in union with the Bishop of Rome.

More germane to the field of Medical Ethics, however, is the exercise of the teaching authority of the Church in other instances, and apart from the charism of infallibility, in the moral teachings of the Roman Pontiff alone, or with the expressed concurrence of the Bishops of the world, as well as the teaching of the individual Bishop in his proper diocese.

The Second Vatican Council likewise spoke clearly to these questions.

In matters of faith and morals, the bishops speak in the name of Christ, and the faithful are to accept their teaching and adhere to it with religious assent of soul. This religious submission of will and of mind must be shown in a special way to the authentic teaching authority of the Roman Pontiff, even when he is not speaking *ex cathedra*. That is, it must be shown in such a way that his supreme magisterium is acknowledged with reverence, the judgments made by him are sincerely adhered to, according to his manifest mind and will. His mind and will in the matter may be known chiefly, either from the character of the documents, from his frequent repetition of the same doctrine, or from his manner of speaking.[8]

The Roman Pontiff exercises the charism of infallibility only when teaching strictly according to the conditions described in the decree of the Vatican Council. Pontifical decrees, instructions, encyclical letters, or pontifical authorization of the decisions of the Sacred Congregations, are not solemn definitions. A respectful internal assent is due such documents, because of the great weight of their authority, but they are not necessarily irreformable, as is a definition.

Moreover, the authoritative force of such papal pronouncements may vary according to the subject matter, the intention of the Roman Pontiff, and the nature and scope of his audience. Encyclicals, radio messages and allocutions, usually contain matter that is considered to be generally as essential to Catholic doctrine. Other statements, which deal directly with questions of morality and are pronounced within the context of the responsibility of the Apostolic See to intervene authoritatively, constitute an integral part of the "ordinary" teaching of the Pope.[9] This is particularly clear when they are spoken to a large professional group and/or, at the direction of the Pope, are published for global communication in the Acts of the Apostolic See. Although not infallible, these statements merit the respect of and acceptance by the faithful.

Natural Law and Divine Law

Intimately bound up with the teaching authority of the Church is the complex notion of law. The terms "natural law" and "divine positive law" have fallen out of fashion and are not as widely discussed even in seminaries and theology schools as they once were. Nevertheless, a clear understanding of the terms is necessary for a proper understanding of the Church documents and magisterial statements that continue to use these concepts to deal with complex human problems.

The distinction "divine" and "natural" here is an artificial one insofar as both types of law have as their origin God. The distinction has arisen in history, however, in order to focus on the *method* that God has used to make His will known to mankind.

The natural law is not to be confused with the physical laws of nature, which are only descriptions of observed constant phenomena in nature, such as the law of gravity. The natural law is understood rather as the design, in nature, that reflects the Creator's will with regard to human fulfillment, as recognized through natural reason.

The founders of American democracy were reflecting the natural law in those words of the Declaration of Independence: "We hold these truths to be self-evident (i.e., learned from natural reason): that all men are created equal (design in nature), and endowed by their Creator with certain unalienable rights (reflecting the Creator's will), etc."

Thomas Aquinas perceived the natural law as God's plan imprinted in man's nature and wrote that "natural law is nothing other than the participation of eternal law in rational creatures."[10] The Fathers of the Second Vatican Council, in their plea to mankind to curb the savagery of war, stated: ". . . the Council wishes to recall first of all the permanent binding force of universal natural law and its all-embracing principles."[11]

The fundamental concept of natural law is inherent in human consciousness, and long antedates what we might call the 2500 year history of western philosophy. And even within those two millennia, from Sophocles to Santayana, the many variations of the basic idea wax and wane through Plato and Aristotle, Paul and Aquinas, and the Post-Reformation modalities of Hugo Grotius, Hobbs, Locke and Kant, and on through our contemporary philosophical mix. While all of this belongs more properly to a History of Philosophy, it is important for us to note here that the Catholic Church discerns within the charism of her teaching authority, the prerogative to illuminate the natural law in the light of that divine assistance promised by Jesus Christ. Indeed this guidance is often needed for an adequate knowledge of the natural law.[12] A frequently overlooked but very important dimension of this illumination of the natural law by the teaching Church, is that for the believing Catholic, the motive of credibility on a given point is not only the force of the natural law argument (which in the nature of the case may be obscure or inconclusive), but likewise the charismatic sacramentality of the Church itself.

The divine positive law, on the other hand, is the divine Will of the Creator made manifest in the messianic revelation of God's Incarnate Word—the teachings of Jesus. The credibility of this law, for all mankind, rests ultimately on supernatural faith. But the reasonable preamble of Christian faith includes an academic evaluation of the genuinity of the documents which report the messianic message, their historical accuracy, and the authenticity of their central figure. Such a preamble developed in the many standard works of fundamental theology.

Canon Law and Civil Law

Besides "natural" and "divine" law, often the notions of "canon" and "civil" law enter into medical moral questions. Canon law is the ecclesial legislation of the Catholic Church, and civil law is the legal regulation of the civic community. Each of these, in itself, is human law, although each may contain by way of reiteration certain elements of divine positive or natural law. Both canon and civil law will receive further attention as the need arises in this work.

CHAPTER TWO

BASIC PRINCIPLES

The following considerations on the nature of law, obligation, and related concepts may, at first glance, seem extraneous to the field of Medical Ethics. Christian morality, however, is a normative science and the norms, as we have seen, are inherent in law. Natural law, divine positive law, canon law and civil law are, after all, only various, more detailed specifications of the universal law of love. Thus an adequate evaluation of many of the questions that arise in medical morality will depend on an understanding of some of the related notions of law and man's response to it.

Law and Obligation

Law is defined as a permanent rational norm for free activity, enacted and adequately promulgated by the one who is in charge of the community, to safeguard and advance the common good, and specified by legitimate authority, as in some way participating in the plan of creation.

A law that is just, useful, possible of observance, and adequately promulgated, gives rise to an obligation in the subjects of the law.

An unjust law would be destructive of right order. A law would be useless if it were without relationship to right order, and its observance would be impossible if it made demands beyond human capacities, or, if it were not adequately made known or promulgated.

The concept of the common good, and its relationship to law and obligation, has always been stressed in philosophical and legal writings. This is because the common good is not only the basic context for the personal fulfillment of the individual, but also is necessarily the immediate concern of civil law, as well as a very useful criterion in seeking to determine some of the more minute refinements of the natural law. However, we must not lose sight of the fact that this is an immediate and practical aspect of law, serving its more ultimate and fundamental purpose, which is the self-realization and fulfillment of the individual.

The common good is meaningless, except in so far as it protects and enhances the good of the individuals, who make up the community, whether that community be the Church, the State, or the World.

And thus although law gives rise to obligation and restriction, the restriction of true obligation is not in the nature of a blockade, which frustrates and thwarts; but rather the restriction of a channel, which gathers up and activates and releases potential power. In man (as well as in the impersonal physical order), unrestricted and undirected energy tends only to dissipate itself without self-realization, and more often than not destroys its own environment. It is the purpose of law, whether natural, divine positive, canon or civil, to protect, direct, and liberate the human thrust toward its own best accomplishment, and its own deepest fulfillment.

Law imposes an obligation which is made immediately effective upon the subject of the law through the medium of conscience. Moral conscience is a judgment of the intellect—or the intellect itself as habitually judging—about the moral goodness or badness of an action. Thus conscience is seen to be the practical rule of action, or the immediate, working norm of morality for every individual. It is to be noted, however, that the individual conscience is not to be understood as a teacher of morality. It is, rather, the individual judgment as to whether or not a specific action is in accord with moral teaching.

Traditionally, conscience has been divided into the categories of *true, erroneous, certain, doubtful,* and *scrupulous.* A true conscience correctly judges the moral quality of an action. It interprets accurately whether or not an action is truly loving and wholesome. An erroneous conscience is a judgment which is not in conformity to objective truth. A certain conscience is a moral judgment which is unaccompanied by any fear of error, since the motive for the judgment is recognized to be sound. A doubtful conscience is had when the intellect suspends judgment as to the moral quality of an action because of insufficient evidence. A scrupulous conscience is characterized by a chronically erroneous manner of judging the morality of actions due to an unreasonable fear of sin.

In the context of these distinctions, it is clear that a certain conscience must always be obeyed, and is required for licit action. A doubtful conscience must be rendered certain in practice, before being used as a norm of action. One may never act in a practical doubt about the morality of an action.

By practical doubt is meant a doubt about the moral goodness or badness of an individual action, here and now, in these particular circumstances. To act in such a doubt is tantamount to accepting evil, since one would be seeking an object, whether the object be morally good, or morally evil.

Most often, a doubt can be resolved by having recourse to well established moral principles. At other times, no certain guidelines can be found to apply to a specific concrete situation. In such an instance, the individual is often faced with a number of options, which are all with solid probability, considered morally acceptable. He is then free to follow the course of action he deems desirable even if some of the other options open to him, objectively speaking, appear to be more probable. The individual is not obliged to follow the most restrictive course of action, since obligation can only be imposed on the individual when there is a certain known moral necessity.

In acting on a moral opinion, however, the individual must be certain that it truly enjoys solid probability. Opinions that go against the clear and explicit teachings of the Church can scarcely be considered to enjoy a solid probability.

This principle of probabilism is derived from an analysis of the nature of obligation. It can be seen in very early theologians, but first received explicit formulation by Bartholomew Medina about 1577. Often it has been misused and misunderstood. In the debates over *Humanae Vitae*, for example, some theologians have misinterpreted this principle. The argument ran as follows. Since some reputable theologians published opinions contrary to the encyclical's teaching on birth control, the issue was in doubt. Since the issue was in a state of irresolvable doubt, the individual was free to follow any probable opinion he deemed desirable in this issue. Since in cases of irresolvable doubt, an individual is not obliged to follow the most restrictive opinion, he could in practice follow the beliefs of the dissenting theologians.

But, the argument is flawed, because of the nature of the material being treated. The encyclical itself makes it clear that the dissenting opinions cannot be held to be solidly probable. Moreover, the Bishops of the United States in their collective pastoral letter, "Human Life in Our Day," offered the following carefully worded analyses of the situation of dissenting from non-infallible doctrine.

When there is question of theological dissent from non-infallible doctrine, we must recall that there is always a presumption in favor of the magisterium. Even non-infallible authentic doctrine, though it may admit of development, or call for clarification or revision, remains binding and carries with it a moral certitude, especially when it is addressed to the universal Church, without ambiguity, in response to urgent questions bound up with faith and crucial to morals. The expressions of theological dissent from the magisterium is in order only if the reasons are serious and well-founded, if the manner of the dissent does not question, or impugn the teaching authority of the Church, and is such, as not to give scandal . . . Even responsible dissent does not excuse one from faithful representation of authentic doctrine of the Church when one is performing a pastoral ministry in her name.

It is clear from the above that in spite of the theological dissent, the bishops did not believe the issue to truly be in doubt but that the encyclical's teaching, although open to clarification, carried with it the weight of "moral certitude."

Subjects of Law

In general, subjects of the law are those over whom the legislator has jurisdiction, and whom he intends to bind. Moreover, since the meaning of law includes the concept of a rational directive of free activity, one must have attained the use of reason in order to be formally a subject of the law.

The natural law obliges all men. Moreover, since the natural law is based on the very fact of existing human nature, it can also be said to oblige even those who have not reached the use of reason. Obviously those who have not reached the use of reason, or those who are perpetually insane, cannot formally violate the natural law. However, they are under the law and are subjects of the law, and therefore, one who would incite them to a material violation of the law, would himself bear the guilt of such a violation.

Divine positive law obliges all those who have attained the use of reason. Purely ecclesiastical laws oblige only the baptized, who have attained the use of reason and have completed their seventh year, unless some other express provision is made.[13]

1. The canons regarding the reception of the sacraments in danger of death, and the precepts of Easter Communion and annual confession declare that the law in these matters binds the faithful who have attained the use of reason, even if they are under the age of seven years.

2. Canons 1099 and 1070 exempt baptized non-Catholics from the canonical form of marriage, and from the invalidating impediment of disparity of cult.

3. Canon 88 prescribes that the habitually insane are to be canonically considered as infants, under the age of seven.

4. Certain canons inflict ecclesiastical penalties (e.g., excommunication) *ipso facto* upon the commission of certain crimes (e.g., abortion). In virtue of canon 2230 those under fourteen years of age are excused from such penalties, but those who induce them to the crime or who canonically cooperate with them, do incur the penalties.

Other Divisions of Law

An affirmative precept of law is one that enjoins that some act be done. A negative precept is one that forbids some act. It is important to note that there can never be an exception or excusing cause from a negative precept of the natural law. The reason for this is evident: a strictly negative precept of the natural law merely delineates some action as being positively destructive of right order, based on the very concept of human nature itself. An affirmative precept, on the other hand, delineates some action as being in accord with right order, or demanded by right order, but not at all times or under all circumstances.

Moral law is a law which imposes an obligation directly in conscience. Whether the moral obligation is grave or light is determined by the nature of the matter enjoined and by the will of the legislator. To establish the gravity of the obligation, it is necessary to consider the nature of the matter, the wording of the law, its object, motive, circumstances, sanction, and usual interpretation.

Penal law imposes an obligation only indirectly in conscience; namely, it imposes an obligation in conscience to acknowledge and accept the just penalty for transgression.

Whether a law imposes a moral or merely a penal obligation depends upon the intention of the legislator and the nature of the law. It is certain that the natural, divine positive, and canon laws impose a moral obligation.

The civil laws, in so far as they are purely civil laws, and not a reiteration of some natural or divine positive law, are considered to be purely penal laws. This doctrine, for the following reasons, is proposed as at least probable in theory, and therefore, certain in practice.

1. From the Intention of the Legislator: It is not to be supposed that the legislator intends to oblige the more conscientious members of a civil society to a moral obligation, when he knows that the same law will not be considered, by a great number of the subjects, as imposing a moral obligation.

2. From the Nature of the Case: In our present civil context it can be proved that purely penal laws are necessary for the common good, but it cannot be proved that it is necessary for purely civil laws to impose a moral obligation,

in order that the common good be safeguarded and advanced.

Any competent authority can legislate invalidating, or incapacitating laws, within the scope of its own authority, whose effect is to render an action, which of its nature would be valid, legally null and void, unless certain conditions are fulfilled. Such laws are sometimes necessary for the common good.

Moreover, it is to be noted that ignorance of the invalidating, or incapacitating law, normally does not prevent the effect of the law.

Observance of Law

Because law is founded upon the necessity of safeguarding and advancing the common good, it is evident that the obligation to observe the law also includes within itself the obligations of taking the ordinary means to know the law, of employing ordinary care to observe the law, of removing or preventing proximate obstacles to the fulfillment of the law, and of avoiding proximate danger of violating the law.

In order to satisfy the obligation of a law, as long as what the law demands is done, neither the intention to accomplish the purpose of the law, nor the intention to satisfy the obligation by this particular act, is required.

A negative precept of law is fulfilled merely by abstaining from the prohibited action.

Cessation of Obligation

It is evident that obligation becomes inoperative in the presence of the impossibility of observing the law. This concept is further refined in the notion of "moral" impossibility. The principle of equity can likewise affect the obligation to observe some laws.

Physical Impossibility: Physical impossibility obviously excuses from the observance of all laws.

Moral Impossibility: Moral impossibility does not mean actual impossibility in the ordinary sense of the word, but refers to those circumstances in which observance of the law would demand something like "heroism beyond the call of duty." Moral impossibility excuses from the observance of any law, except the negative precepts of the natural law.

This is because the negative precepts of the natural law forbid only what is intrinsically evil, such as idolatry, blasphemy, perjury, onanism, etc. Such things are not to be admitted, even at the cost of life itself. Because the preservation of human life is not man's ultimate end, but man has further and higher goals, right order can sometimes demand the sacrifice of even life itself.

Regarding moral impossibility in the observance of other kinds of law, the effort required to constitute moral impossibility, which might range in a particular case from grave inconvenience to heroism, is to be judged in proportion to the importance of the law, i.e., the good to be achieved by its observance.

Epikeia (equity): Epikeia, or equity, is an interpretation of the law in a particular case, the interpretation being against the letter of the law, but in accord with its spirit and the reasonably presumed mind of the legislator.

The reasonableness of *epikeia* is based on the presumption that the legislator, in framing the law, cannot foresee all circumstances, but envisions only the ordinary contingencies and would wish his law to be humanely administered. Thus, obviously, *epikeia* does not apply to the natural law.

Voluntariety and the Human Act

A human person is a dynamism, constantly in action. The first distinction we observe in these actions is that some of them are had in common with other living things (e.g., metabolism, sensation, etc.), and some of them are specifically human (e.g., intellection and free will). These latter types of action, which belong uniquely to man and are specifically human, are known as "human acts." And of these specifically human acts, those which are deliberate acts of the free will, and for which, therefore, man is morally responsible, are called "voluntary acts."

Voluntary Act: A voluntary act is a deliberate action of man's free will, placed with knowledge and advertence.

To be perfectly and specifically voluntary, the act must be

an act which the will places freely, with antecedent knowledge of its moral object, motive, and circumstances, and with accompanying advertence.

Determining Elements of a Voluntary Act: The triple complexus of moral object, motive and circumstance constitute the determining elements of a voluntary act. Within them is found that mixture of real and apparent good, which is represented to the will, and in regard to which the will makes its free choice.

These are what we might call the elemental constituents of the morality of any human action, because an action is morally good or morally bad in so far as these elements are, or are not, in accord with right order. A more detailed treatment of these three elements is necessary, because it is frequently only by analyzing a situation under these three aspects that we can form a correct moral judgment.

Moral Object: This is the most difficult to understand of the three determinants. Briefly, the moral object is that to which the will immediately and primarily directs itself.

It is extremely important to remember here that we are dealing with the moral order, and therefore we are speaking of the moral object of an action, and not merely the physical or ontological object.

If I think of an action merely as walking, eating, drinking, shooting, etc., I am thinking of a purely ontological, or physical object of the will, because these things, as such, have not yet acquired any relation to the moral order. A moral object would be blasphemy, adultery, or theft.

For example, in an act of theft we can distinguish:

1. The taking away of something;
2. That belongs to another;
3. Against his will;
4. When his unwillingness is reasonable.

In the foregoing analysis of an act of theft, numbers 1, 2, and 3, (the taking away of something, that belongs to another, against his will), considered alone, represent nothing in the moral order. Such an act might be good, or it might be bad. Number 4, however (when his unwillingness is reasonable), gives the act a moral complexion, and identifies the act as "theft." Theft is the moral object.

Circumstances: In the above example, number 4 is actually a circumstance that gives the act any relation at all to the moral order, i.e., the first circumstance that takes the act out of the merely physical order and puts it into the moral order. We include such a circumstance under the moral object.

Other circumstances, which we might call aggravating or mitigating circumstances, can change the gravity of this particular moral object, as for example the circumstance of "how much" or "from whom." Thus aggravating or mitigating circumstances can make the moral object more or less serious. Still other circumstances might actually add a new moral object.

Motive: Motive is really a circumstance too, but since it is the first element in determining a free act of the will, it is considered separately.

A human act is said to be a morally good act if its moral object, motive(s) and circumstances are all in accord with right order. An act is identified as morally bad if one or more of these determinants is in serious conflict with right order.

Human motivation, of course, is not always simple. We are all familiar with the expression "mixed motives." In this summary it is sufficient to point out that a secondary and slightly compromised additional motive would not destroy the moral goodness of a properly motivated and otherwise morally good act, although it would obviously affect it in some way. The same may be said of a minor defect of circumstances.[14]

These considerations bring up the familiar question of whether "the end justifies the means?" We will pass over the 19th century controversy arising out of the absurd charge of Blaise Pascal that the Jesuits taught that a good end justifies an evil means, a false charge that was ultimately settled by the Court of Appeals of Cologne in 1903. The answer, of course, is "yes" in the sense that normally the means one takes to accomplish a good work may be said to participate in the goodness of the end. It is "no" in the sense that a morally wrong act does not become good because it is done for a good end or purpose.

Current problems regarding euthanasia highlight this concept. Contrary to Catholic teaching, Joseph Fletcher would hold that in some circumstances the direct killing of a terminal patient (means) would be morally justified by the intended consequences (end) of the act of killing; such as to save the expenses of terminal care, to alleviate the anxiety of the family, to put the patient out of his misery, etc. Commenting on such a case, Fletcher writes: "The priority of the end is paired with the 'principle of proportionate good'; any disvalue in the means must be outweighed by the value gained in the end . . . It comes down to this, that in some situations a morally good end can justify a relatively 'bad' means, on the principle of proportionate good."[15] This, we believe, is the central error of Fletcher's situation ethic.

Obstacles to Voluntariety

In the moral order a man is responsible for only his specifically human actions. Anything, therefore, that impairs the voluntariety of these actions by impairing the elements of knowledge or freedom in the action, alters the imputability of the action to the degree to which the voluntariety is lessened. Ignorance, error, fear, concupiscence, and habit are considered here as the usual obstacles to complete voluntariety.

Ignorance and Error: In the final analysis one chooses not necessarily what a thing is in itself, but rather what one perceives or judges it to be. The act of the will is ultimately determined by the object as the intellect represents it. For example, if a man sees a coin in a blind beggar's cup, and thinks that the coin is a penny, whereas it is really a five dollar gold piece; stealing it, his act, though physically is the taking of a five dollar gold piece, morally is the stealing of a penny.

Invincible Ignorance: Invincible ignorance is ignorance which cannot be corrected by reasonable diligence. Such an ignorance of the objective morality of an act excuses from all imputability.

Vincible Ignorance: Vincible ignorance is ignorance which could be corrected by reasonable diligence. We have seen that if there is a reasonable possibility of solving a moral doubt by means of study or inquiry, this must be done. It is only after this possibility has been evacuated that one can legitimately deduce a certain practical judgment from the principles of probabilism. And so, regarding an action placed in consciously neglected ignorance, one is morally guilty to the degree to which he sees the obligation to inquire, and fails to fulfill it.

Fear and Concupiscence: Mental anxiety in the face of an impending evil (fear), or movements of the sensitive appetite responding to the imagination (concupiscence), likewise sometimes tend to impair the freedom of the will; but they decrease imputability only to the extent to which they actually do impair that freedom.

It should be noted particularly, with regard to fear and concupiscence, that although these decrease imputability or guilt, one must not necessarily conclude that a person acting under these influences cannot be guilty of grave sin.

Guilt is not notably reduced by fear or concupiscence, unless these influences so disturb the mental equilibrium that the individual almost ceases to be the master of his own actions. An action might be performed under pressure of great fear, and still be a perfectly free act.

Of these two, concupiscence is more apt to obscure the equilibrium of the moral judgment than is fear. In either case, before guilt is greatly reduced, the agent must be so subjectively disturbed that his moral judgment can be compared to that of a man half-asleep, or partially intoxicated: the mind being so disturbed that the avoidance of wrongdoing although physically possible, would exceed the ordinary capacity of men.

Habit: That facility of acting which is acquired by repeated acts (habit), does decrease the imputability of the habitual act, in so far as it decreases freedom and advertence. However, the obligation to rid oneself of the bad habit remains.

Pathologic Obstacles: Aside from a consideration of these normal obstacles to freedom, one should be aware of the way in which freedom is influenced by the various psychic disorders such as schizophrenia, neurasthenia, hysteria, compulsion phenomena, melancholia, etc. In many cases certain images so take possession of the mind that the individual cannot attend to other considerations, or can do so only with great difficulty, and consequently freedom and imputability are either altogether lost, or diminished to a greater or lesser degree.

Principle of the Double Effect

The principle of double effect is merely an analytical approach to a problem which enters, to a greater or lesser degree, into practically every human act. Normally the problem is so slight that it is solved by the simplest act of the moral conscience. But in some situations a more clearly elaborated analysis of the principle is needed in order to evaluate a given action in its relation to right order.

The Problem: No human act is a completely closed, controlled, and independent unit. Any human act, although placed for some particular purpose (motive), and aimed at some particular good (moral object), has a myriad diversity of other effects and repercussions, in one's own life, and in the lives of others, which may be foreseen to some extent, even though not directly intended or willed.

Example: John, the administrator of a private hospital, employs Bertha, an extremely efficient and quite indispensable head nurse, who is not only somewhat temperamental, but likewise careless in some few procedures. For the good of the hospital John must rectify Bertha's carelessness. He knows that to do this he must give her a severe reprimand. He likewise knows that this will result in the correction of her carelessness. But also he is quite sure that, as an added result of his action, the temperamental Bertha will indulge in alcoholic beverages on her next week-end to the extent of objectively serious moral disorder.

Thus the problem: When an action will have two effects, one good effect which is intended, and another evil effect which is foreseen, not, however, as intended but only as permitted, it is evident that the agent is in some way responsible for both effects. It is his action which does produce the two effects, and if he did not place the action, the evil effect would not materialize here and now.

The question therefore arises: Does right order demand that one refrain from such an action; and, if not, under what circumstances is such an action consonant with right order?

In approaching the answer to this question we must recall that man's responsibility for the fundamental tenet of the natural law (i.e., that right order must be preserved), immediately imposes upon him two basic and fundamental obligations:

1. Man must not intend to do that which is evil. (It is to be noted that this is a negative precept of the natural law.)
2. Man must prevent evil in so far as he can reasonably do so. (This is an affirmative precept.)

We have already seen that an affirmative precept does not constitute an unlimited obligation. In other words, there can be circumstances which excuse from the obligation of an affirmative precept.

In the ordinary course of our lives, we constantly find ourselves in the position of wishing to do something which is good in itself, and which will achieve some desired and intended good effect. All other things being equal, there is no reason why we should not go ahead and perform such an action. For example, a doctor may wish to surgically remove the cancerous cervix of a fifty-year-old woman.

Sometimes, however, "all other things" are not equal. We will sometimes foresee that an act, good in itself, and while producing the good effect which we rightfully intend and desire, will also, as a sort of by-product, produce an evil effect, neither desired nor intended, but clearly foreseen. For example, a doctor may wish to remove the cancerous cervix of a twenty-five-year-old woman who is also pregnant. Obviously, in addition to the removal of the cancerous tissue, fetal death is going to result.

In such circumstances there can be no question of intending the evil effect. But this question does arise: "Does the obligation to prevent evil oblige one to abstain from a good action, in order to prevent the concomitant evil, which is foreseen but merely permitted?"

Briefly, the answer is this: one can be obliged only to take reasonable means to prevent evil. Hence, all things considered, if the intended good effect is so great that its omission would be, in the judgment of prudent men, too high a price to pay for the preventing of the concomitant evil, then there is no obligation to abstain from the good action and sacrifice its good effect in order to prevent the concomitant evil.

The Principle of Double Effect: An action, good in itself, which has two effects, an intended and otherwise not reasonably attainable good effect, and foreseen but merely permitted concomitant evil effect, may licitly be placed, provided there is a due proportion between the intended good and the permitted evil.

Because a large proportion of the problems arising in medical-moral considerations are solved by the principle of double effect, we will now investigate each of the key words of the principle, in order to arrive at a concise understanding of this important matter.

An action: Since we are dealing here with the question of the morality of an action, the action is understood to be a specifically human action, placed freely and with advertence.

Good in itself: The action, in itself, and considered apart from the concomitant evil effect, must be a morally good, or at least indifferent action.

Which has two effects: Both the good and the evil effects are actually results of the action in question.

An intended good effect: The intended good effect is called the "direct voluntary." It is the good which really determines the will to act.

Otherwise not reasonably attainable: If the good effect could be obtained in some other way, equally expeditious and effective, and without the concomitant evil effect, obviously this would have to be done. In such a case there would be no proportionate reason for permitting the evil effect.

And a merely permitted evil effect: This is called the "indirect voluntary," that is, although it is foreseen as an evil effect resulting from the action, it is in no way an object of the will act. Its only connection with the will is indirect, and in this way: that the act which is the will-object does in some way cause the evil effect.

Here we must distinguish carefully between moral and physical evil. We are speaking of an evil effect in the moral order only. The evil effect is that which, if directly willed, would be morally evil.

For example, contrast the amputation of a gangrenous leg with the death of a non-viable fetus. In the former case the loss of the leg is a physically, but not morally, evil effect. The leg, as a part of the whole body, is subordinated to the good of the whole. In this case the amputation, although a physical evil, is not a moral evil, if directly willed.

In the latter case, however, granted a cancer of the cervix with a non-viable fetus in situ, the surgeon intends the removal of dangerously diseased tissue. He foresees that the result of his attaining this good effect will be fetal death. He does not seek, intend, or directly will fetal death, but merely foresees it. If he directly willed fetal death, his action would be morally evil.

May licitly be placed: i.e., without moral guilt.

Provided there is due proportion between the intended and the pemitted evil: It would obviously be contrary to right order to permit some very serious damage as a secondary result of an action whose good effect would be relatively insignificant.

This due proportion between the good intended and the evil permitted, is not something that can be measured exactly. It is rather a matter of prudent human judgment.

Summary: In attempting to solve a case under the principle of double effect, the following five points should be checked in each particular set of circumstances.

1. That the action, in itself, be good or at least indifferent.
2. That the good effect cannot be obtained in some equally expeditious and effective way, without the concomitant evil effect.
3. That the evil effect be not directly willed, but only permitted. Under no condition can the action be even partially prompted by a desire for the evil effect. Otherwise

the evil effect becomes a direct voluntary.

4. That the evil effect be not a means to producing the good effect; because if the evil effect is a means to producing the good effect, then the evil effect, like any other means, is necessarily directly willed.

5. That there be a due proportion between the good that is intended and the evil that is permitted.

The Principles of Cooperation

As the concept is analyzed in moral theology, "cooperation" is understood to mean the participation of more than one person in the same immoral, or criminal action. Circumstances may arise in which a man is associated, to a greater or lesser degree, with someone else in a situation which is contrary to right order. Such an associate may be equally guilty with the wrongdoer, or less guilty, or perhaps not guilty at all.

There are any number of examples of this in medical practice. It is clear, for instance, that the surgeon who kills an unborn baby (abortion), is guilty of a serious breach of the moral law. But what about his assistant at the operation, or his anesthetist, both of whom are cooperating in the operation?

In order to judge clearly the existence or degree of guilt in such cooperation, it is necessary to define the various kinds of cooperation, and then to establish some principles regarding them.

Formal Cooperation: Formal cooperation is had whenever one takes some part in the immoral action of another, while at the same time adopting the evil intention of his associate. Thus if the intention of the anesthetist is the same as the intention of the surgeon in an illicit operation (for example, to perform a contraceptive sterilization), the cooperation of the anesthetist is called formal cooperation. Formal cooperation in the sinful act of another is always wrong, and the cooperator is equally guilty with the principal agent, because the will of each of them is determined by the same evil.

Immediate Material Cooperation: Immediate material cooperation is had when one person actually performs the immoral action in cooperation with another person.

Thus, in the operation referred to above, if the surgeon and the assistant are both engaged in actually aborting the fetus, the cooperation of the assistant is said to be immediate material cooperation, because he is doing the actual abortion with the surgeon.

Immediate material cooperation in the sinful act of another is always wrong, and the cooperator is equally guilty with the principal agent, because they both actually do the wrongdoing. Immediate material cooperation is also necessarily formal cooperation because it is vacuous to say that a person in his right senses performs a criminal action without intending, in his will, to do so.[16]

Mediate Material Cooperation: Mediate material cooperation is concurrence in the sinful action of another, not however in such a way that one actually places the act with the other, or concurs in the evil intention of the other; but while merely doing something which is good or indifferent in itself, actually does also supply an occasion of sin to another; or supplies some assistance, means, or preparation for the sinful action of another.

In the case of mediate material cooperation, as far as the will of the cooperator is concerned, it is not so much that one is cooperating in the sin of another, as that the other person is using the good or indifferent action of the cooperator as an occasion of, or assistance to his crime.

Therefore, since the mediate cooperator foresees, but does not intend, this added result of his action, it is evident that he is faced with a problem which falls under the principle of double effect.

The morality of mediate material cooperation is to be sought in the principle of double effect, with special attention to the proportion between the cooperation (how proximate or remote, how necessary or unnecessary, to the crime of another), and the gravity of the crime in connection with which another will make use of it.

In evaluating mediate material cooperation by the principle

of double effect, and in judging the proportion between the gravity of the evil effect, and the proximity and necessity of the cooperation, several important points must be kept in mind.

1. The good effect will be, at least, my own freedom of action, plus the value to me of doing this or that action, not wrong in itself. For example, administering an anesthetic is an indifferent action. For a resident in Anesthesiology to administer anesthesia during an abortion, even though under duress, might represent for him the continuation of this particular residency training program.

2. The evil effect will usually have a double aspect. First there is the fact that my action constitutes an occasion of sin for someone else, or at least an assistance to his crime; and secondly there may be the consideration of some evil coming upon a third party as the result of my action.

It is evident that both of these effects are evil, because they are both contrary to that law of well-ordered love, which is the foundation of all inter-personal morality.

Example: A pregnant mother is psychiatrically ill enough to want someone to kill her baby before it is born. Let us say that this will require the services of a staff obstetrician and a resident anesthetist; and that the anesthetist, envisioning the ideal of his medical practice as the protection of life, is totally unwilling to cooperate, although his professional future may be compromised by this stand.

Administering the anesthesia is not the same as doing the abortion. Thus his cooperation is not *formal*, but *mediate material* cooperation. The good effect will be the protection of his medical career. The evil effects will be all the violations of the law of love that are involved in the situation. Assisting another in any immoral action is a disservice to the other, and this contrary to well-ordered love of one's neighbor. And in this case, since the act is an abortion, there is likewise an appalling lack of love for the infant who is to be killed. Thus the resident feels that he shouldn't be rendering even an ancillary service in such a situation. But then again what about so many others who are somehow in on it, whether they want to be or not? There are the surgical nurses, and the floor nurse who preps the patient, and the orderly who wheels her to the surgical unit, etc.

If the refusal of the anesthetist to cooperate would prevent the abortion, it is difficult to see how he could agree to do so under any circumstances. In the usual case, however, someone else would step in and the operation would proceed without him. If he does cooperate, what is the extent of his responsibility for the evils that ensue? He is not responsible for the obstetrician's own personality distortion (i.e., in this case, "*sin*"), because that has already been determined. He does not abort the baby, and indeed he is against that, but he allows his talents to be used in these undesirable adjuncts. What then is the interplay of culpability and co-responsibility? "

From an analysis of the foregoing example we can discern the differences among the various kinds of mediate material cooperation. *Proximate material cooperation:* administering the anesthesia. *Remote material cooperation:* the routine functions of the floor nurse. *Necessary material cooperation:* administering the anesthetic in the supposition that there is not another anesthetist available. *Non-necessary material cooperation:* administering the anesthetic in the supposition that there is another anesthetist, either at hand or available, who would administer the anesthetic anyhow.

Principles:

1. Mediate material cooperation in a serious evil, which is also proximate cooperation, is permitted only if necessary to escape a very serious damage.
2. Mediate material cooperation in a serious evil, which is also necessary cooperation, is permitted only if necessary to escape a very serious damage.
3. Mediate material cooperation in a serious evil, which is both proximate and necessary cooperation, is permitted only if necessary to escape an extremely serious damage.

    Moreover, in a case in which there is question of serious harm to a third party and the cooperation is both proximate and truly necessary (so that the harm to the third party would not happen if cooperation were withheld), one could offer such cooperation, if, by refusing his cooperation, he would suffer damage commensurable to the foreseen harm to the third party. The law of charity imposes this more definitive restriction only where the cooperation is both proximate and necessary. But even here charity does not oblige one to prevent harm to a third party when, in doing so, one would himself suffer an equal harm.

4. Mediate material cooperation, which is non-necessary and very remote, is permitted for a reasonable cause.

5. In other cases the degree of necessity or proximity of the cooperation must be judged in proportion to the evil effect, and in proportion to the advantage the cooperator will find in the good effect, in order to arrive at an honest estimate of how serious a reason one must have to cooperate in a particular evil action.

Negative Cooperation

Negative cooperation is understood as cooperation in the sin of another by neglecting to do something which obliges either by office or position. Negative cooperation may be formal or material, and its morality is to be judged according to the principles delineated above.

Particular Cases of Cooperation

It would be impossible to list all the types of problems in cooperation, which might arise in the medical profession. And each case may vary somewhat due to the particular circumstances in which it occurs. The following examples represent some of the more usual types of problems that arise.

The problems most frequently occur in the area of obstetrics, gynecology, and family planning. These are not the only problems, or even the most difficult ones; but it would be less than realistic to pretend that they are not the most frequent problems.

House Officers: An intern or resident physician in a nonsectarian hospital may find that he is expected to take part in certain procedures, which conflict with his ethical principles. The house officer should first clearly determine, in his own mind, what actions are part of the illicit procedure itself (such as ligations and curettage in some cases), and what actions can be described as mediate material cooperation (such as anesthesia, preparatory surgical procedures, or other procedures which do not, of themselves, relate to the illicit action).

Participation in the illicit procedures themselves is never consistent with ethical integrity. In deciding the licitness of mediate material cooperation, it should be remembered that such cooperation should always be under protest, and that the protest must be expressed or at least implied; and if reasonably possible such cooperation should be avoided completely. On the other hand, to seriously compromise one's position in a training program can mean serious damage to one's career. However, experience indicates that a chief, who does not respect the ethical principles of a trainee, is extremely rare. Moreover, in weighing the reasons in favor of undertaking such a program, the good influence, which can be expected from the presence of so sincerely ethical a physician, is not to be overlooked.

Contraceptive Procedures: There is no excuse for a Catholic physician to have anything at all to do with procedures which are directly contraceptive. Grave scandal is caused by a Catholic doctor who, in any way, temporizes in this matter. He cannot, without serious moral guilt, advise or recommend contraception to any patient, no matter what the patient's personal convictions may be. Neither may he instruct a patient in the use of contraception, nor refer the patient to any other physician or agency for this purpose, without seriously compromising his own moral integrity.

Certifying for Therapeutic Abortion: In circumstances where certain conditions are described as "medical" indications for therapeutic abortion, and the abortion cannot be performed unless several physicians certify that these conditions are present, the question may arise as to whether or not a physician may so certify under the supposition that he is merely stating that certain conditions are verified, irrespective of any medical, or moral convictions about therapeutic abortion. Although some moralists have speculated that such restricted certification could be merely mediate material cooperation in the abortion, it is difficult to see how this could be done by an honest man without an intention that would make the cooperation formal. Moreover, grave scandal would preclude the possibility of such certification.

Group Practice: Three questions ordinarily arise in the mind of a Catholic physician contemplating group practice with other physicians who do not accept his medical moral code. There is the question of division of funds wherein the Catholic physician feels that he is profiting financially from certain illicit procedures of his colleagues. Since such a physician would be doing basically his share of the work, and receiving his share of the profits, there is no moral difficulty here.

The second question concerns referrals. As previously pointed out, the sincere Catholic physician could not refer patients to his partners, nor to any other colleagues, for illicit procedures, and still maintain his own intellectual honesty.

The third question is that of scandal. If such a physician is in group practice with others who perform therapeutic abortions, contraceptive sterilizations, etc., he will necessarily appear to approve these procedures, or at least not to seriously disapprove of them. Since, as a physician, he is a leader in the community and looked upon with admiration and respect, his entering such a group practice could tend to weaken the moral stamina of the community, and hence would be morally questionable.

One of the most acute problems regarding cooperation is the broader question of Catholic institutional policy in permitting Catholic health facilities to be used for contraceptive sterilization and abortion. This controversial question became focused after the Bishops of the United States approved the most recent Ethical and Religious Directives for Catholic Health Facilities in November 1971, with the prescriptions of the preamble that: "Any facility identified as Catholic, assumes with this identification the responsibility to reflect in its policies and practices, the moral teachings of the Church, under the guidance of the local

Bishop," and ". . . its [the health facility] Board of Trustees, acting through its chief executive officer, carry an overriding responsibility in conscience to prohibit those procedures, which are morally and spiritually harmful."

This official stand against material cooperation by the Catholic health facility in practices contrary to Catholic teaching was quickly met by an organized opposition within Catholic theological circles. The basic thesis of the opposition was that because a Catholic hospital is really a community facility in a pluralistic society and supported in great part by public funds, it has no right to refuse medical procedures, which although contrary to Catholic teaching, are accepted both medically and ethically by a large segment of the physician-patient community.

This opposition to the policy of the Bishops is, however, afflicted with three glaring inconsistencies. First, most of those Catholics who oppose the Bishops' negative policy on material cooperation would favor contraceptive procedures in Catholic hospitals, but would oppose abortions, although their reasons for allowing contraception would apply equally to abortion. Secondly, they emphasize the exigencies of living in a pluralistic society as though pluralism meant a common morality, whereas it really means the co-existence of varying theological attitudes (including that of the Catholic hospital). Finally, there is neither a moral nor a legal obligation to abandon one's religious principles on the receipt of public funds. This, indeed, has been indicated by federal legislation, which protects certain hospitals (and personnel) benefitting from federal funding from being coerced into performing abortion or sterilization procedures.[17]

The Professional Office Building of A Catholic Hospital

Questions have been raised regarding the propriety of (and regulation of) professional office buildings owned by, and adjacent to, Catholic hospitals vis a vis the Ethical and Religious Directives for Catholic Health Facilities. Prescinding from the proper legal arrangements, the question is one of responsibility and material cooperation.

In one sense, the owner of a professional office building

provides no more than office space to physicians, and this for a price. The physician provides his own equipment, hires his own personnel, keeps his own accounts and, briefly, is his own boss. On the level of cooperation and responsibility, it is evident that the hospital administration would not be as intimately involved with practices contrary to its ethical code by physicians in a corporately owned office building, as by using the hospital facilities for such practices. Yet it would be clearly incorrect to say that the hospital administration bears no responsibility at all for what is done under such an arrangement.

But the real issue of morally unacceptable practices in such an office building would seem to be one of scandal, not in the sense of conduct that is shocking or surprising to others, but rather of conduct that is an occasion of spiritual harm to others. Scandal in this latter sense would be given (to take an extreme but illustrative example), if a religious community or a diocese rented a facility to someone using it as a house of prostitution. Although this might not lead many otherwise good people into the sin of prostitution, it could easily cause disillusion with religion among many, with the consequent neglect of their religious lives and spiritual harm to themselves. On the other hand, if a religious community or a diocese owned an apartment building and rented an apartment to a couple involved in an invalid marriage, the danger of scandal would be obviously less, at least in most cases. Thus the danger of scandal will vary according to the circumstances.

So likewise in the case of the hospital-owned professional office building, the problem must be assessed according to the circumstances of the individual case. Much would depend, for instance, on what kind of violations of the ethical code were in question. If doctors were procuring early abortion in these offices, or performing contraceptive sterilizations, or operating a birth control clinic, the scandal could be very serious if the public were to have the even mistaken impression that this was part of the operation of the Catholic hospital, or being done with the approval, or even positive tolerance of the Catholic hospital.

This danger of scandal and spiritual harm to others should not be considered lightly, but weighed seriously against the advantages of having such a facility. The main advantage to the hospital is likely to be financial, but unless the financial exigency would be imperative even for the survival of the institution, it seems less than appropriate for a religious community, vowed to poverty, to risk spiritual harm to the people of God for financial considerations.

It would be ideal, of course, if all the physicians observed the Catholic institution directives in such offices, and indeed the hospitals should strive to arrange for this in its contractual agreements. But if it cannot be achieved, the alternative is not necessarily to abandon the idea of a professional office building. The circumstances may be such that a less radical solution would be possible, but the goal should always be only to advance the ideal of a Catholic health facility: i.e., to give "witness to the saving presence of Christ and His Church. . ." (cf. Preamble, *Ethical and Religious Directives for Catholic Health Facilities*).

CHAPTER THREE

HUMAN LIFE–RESPONSIBILITY AND RIGHT

Principle of the Inviolability of Human Life

The fundamental explanation of the inviolability of human life arises spontaneously from the previous considerations regarding the existence of God and the nature of man.

One of the most familiar enunciations of this aspect of the natural law is found in our American Declaration of Independence, where this truth is said to be self evident: namely, that "all men are created equal."

This fundamental equality of all men has a very particular meaning. Obviously all men are not created equal in size, or talents, or physical ability, etc., but all men are created equal in this: that they all have the same final destiny and are all equal in their intrinsic dignity as human beings and in their subordination to the creator, and in the rights and duties which this equality and subordination imply.

In the very order of nature, plant life and animal life are subordinated to man, and it is only through man and his use of these things that they can actually fulfill their role in the plan of creation. That is why we can kill a cow and eat it; its final purpose of existence is subordinated to ours. Such things as cabbages and cows are meant to be used by man in order to help man fulfill his destiny.

These fundamental notions of equality and subordination in the order of nature are not easily explored in a few words. They suggest an analysis of rights and duties, the limitations of exercise and control, the individual's proper scope and range of self-determination and relationships to other people and things. It may be helpful to sum this up in the word prerogative, distinguishing between *prerogatives* which are *absolute* in the sense of unrestricted and prerogatives which are "for use only."

One is said to have absolute prerogative in a thing when it is essentially subordinated to one's final end, and has become the object of one's lawful rights.

Thus a man can have an absolute prerogative in his own property or livestock. Its final purpose is subordinated to, and ordered toward, man's final end, and man may use it as a mere means to his own purposes, even to the extent of destroying the substance.

Prerogative for use, on the other hand, is that restricted power or prerogative which a man has, whereby he has some right to use the thing, but with certain restrictions, which are imposed by the higher rights of others.

Thus if a man lends me his car or his horse, I may rightfully use it, but I cannot destroy it for my own purposes, because his title to ownership gives him a prior right to the thing.

A subordination of final ends implies absolute prerogative, whereas an equality of final ends admits of only a prerogative for use.

Prerogative in Human Life

In the light of these considerations it is evident that man can have, at most, only a useful prerogative over human life.

I may hire another man to work for me and use his labor for my own purposes, but I cannot destroy him for my own ends, thus relegating him to the position of being a mere means to my own end.

The other man is ultimately and essentially my equal, and his final end is not subordinated to, but equal to, mine. In this respect he is subordinated to God alone.

Thus when we are dealing with human life—one's own life or the life of another—we are dealing with something in which man can have, at most, only use and stewardship, as a right and responsibility. Absolute prerogative in human life is an exclusively divine prerogative, and right reason demands that any invasion or diminution of human life be considered in the light of this exclusively divine prerogative.

The physician must always remember that the lives and the bodies of his patients are not subordinated to himself, nor to the state, nor to the science of medicine, nor even to the patient himself. They are subordinated to God alone.

The patient is the administrator of his own life and faculties, with only an administrative or useful prerogative, exercising a kind of stewardship. The physician, in his professional relationship, becomes the skilled agent of the patient in this role.

Most of the moral problems presented in contemplated medical procedures can be measured by this rule: Is the contemplated act one of ownership, or of wise stewardship?

The Physician's Delegated Prerogative

Concomitant with the concept of the individual as enjoying an administrative role in his own case, is the concept of the authority of a physician over his patient as an authority delegated to him by the patient.

A patient is an individual who has the right and obligation to preserve his health and bodily integrity. Since, however, in many cases, he does not have the skill or ability to do this himself, he engages one who does have such a skill and ability (a doctor), and delegates to the doctor his own administrative role. The physician has a right to act only within the limits of this delegation; and therefore he must have, in some way, the consent of his patient for whatever he does.

Pius XII expressed this thought most explicitly when speaking of the morality of medical experimentation. The same words, however, are applicable to any physician-patient relationship. "In the first place, it must be assumed that, as a private person, the doctor can take no measure or try no course of action without the consent of his patient. The doctor has no other rights or power over the patient than those which the latter gives him explicitly or implicitly and tacitly."[18]

Implicit Consent of the Patient: As indicated in the passage just quoted, there are times when the actions of the patient or the exigencies of the circumstances allow for the tacit or presumed consent of the patient for certain procedures.

By merely entering into the patient-physician relationship, consent is implied for the customary diagnostic and therapeutic procedures in common use.

Secondly, the unconscious patient's consent for needed therapy, or even surgery, is readily presumed in some circumstances. This might occur in the case of the individual who is found in an unconscious state. It might occur during an operation for which general consent has already been granted, but during which the need for more extensive surgery becomes apparent. We are explicitly dealing only with the basic moral question. Legal complications are best precluded by appropriate release forms.

Thirdly, when it is evident to the physician that a certain treatment is indicated, but the patient is in such a disturbed state of mind as to unreasonably refuse such treatment, the physician may, in some circumstances, presume the rational consent of the patient. The most obvious case of this is the attempted suicide, who refuses the medical attention required to save his life. Another instance could be found in the psychiatric patient, who needs therapeutic measures which he resists. In these instances, the reasonable consent of the patient can in some cases be presumed. The consent of the next of kin should likewise be sought, but sometimes this too might have to be presumed, in the event of their unreasonable resistance. In such cases the physician should be careful that legal requirements are fulfilled.

Before such presumption it should be clear, however, that the particular therapy is critically needed and that the restrictions of the civil law are allowed for.

Fourthly, in dealing with minors, the consent of the older type child, as well as the consent of the parent or guardian, should be obtained. We believe, however, that the refusal of consent by a more advanced minor (e.g., one who could earn his own living), must be respected, whereas in the case of younger children, parental consent is sufficient.

Finally, consideration must be given to the case wherein

necessary treatment is refused by the patient, because of subjectively sincere considerations, which the physician cannot accept as reasonable. In general, as far as the individual patient is concerned, the physician may try to persuade the patient to accept the treatment; but not to force it upon the patient, nor institute such procedures after the patient has lost consciousness. This would be a violation of the rights of the individual patient, unless such procedures were to be demanded for the protection of the common good. The difficult case of the Jehovah's Witness who refuses blood transfusion, even as life-saving procedure, is treated in detail later in this chapter.

The Duty to Preserve Life

Bearing in mind the previously delineated principles regarding the inviolability of human life, and man's administrative role in his own substance, we will now consider several particular problems relating to the preservation of human life. Such clear-cut violations of God's absolute dominion, as euthanasia and suicide, need little elaboration. Other more involved problems, such as the prolongation of life in terminal illness, human experimentation, and clinical research will be treated in greater detail.

Euthanasia and Suicide

The Catholic Church has consistently taught that suicide is a totally undefensible and gravely sinful injection of disordered self-referenced determination into the providential plan of God's love. It is seen as the ultimate violation of the divine prerogative of the author of life. We might add that the divinely endowed rights which the Founding Fathers of American democracy held to be self-evident—such as, first and foremost, the right to life—carry with them certain corresponding fundamental responsibilities. The most profound of these responsibilities is drastically and definitely abandoned in the act of self-destruction, and, indeed, in this context euthanasia and suicide are very much of a piece, and present the same theological distortion of right order.

Ecclesiastical Penalty : According to the provisions of Church law (Canons 1240 and 2350) those who kill themselves "of deliberate purpose" are to be deprived of Christian burial. In view of the norms of canonical interpretation, it is to be noted that when public scandal can be avoided, the penalty is not to be inflicted, unless it is clear that the crime was "of deliberate purpose" and "notorious."

Such deliberateness, notoriety, and scandal will be rare, while the more or less common opinion prevails that suicide usually results from mental derangement.

The physician will frequently be asked to give an opinion in this matter, and he should not do so lightly, but should remember the serious implications of the fact that ecclesiastical procedure in a very delicate matter will be based, in a large measure, upon his opinion.

Prolongation of Life in Terminal Illness

One of the most difficult problems facing the physician today is the question of prolongation procedures in terminal illness. The question, of course, does not arise in all cases of terminal illness. But there are circumstances in which the conscientious doctor wonders how long he must or should battle imminent dissolution with the array of modern medical and surgical aids and techniques at his disposal.

What, for example, is to be done in regard to the patient dying of advanced carcinoma and in terminal coma, being kept alive by every possible means, while the expense is impoverishing his family? What of the infant with a negative prognosis in spina bifida, and encephalitis who develops pneumonia? Should penicillin be administered and what are the moral dimensions of such questions?

We have already indicated the ultimate parameters of man's stewardship, and the fundamental rights and responsibilities, which are his as the object of creative Love.

Yet the fundamental dynamism of human life implies a process of continual breaking down and building up, an expenditure and restoration of energy, an attrition and repair of the cellular system, which make certain forms of neglect tantamount to self-destruction.

Thus it is evident that the refusal of the everyday means of sustaining life, such as nutrition, rest, and relaxation, is, in effect, a self-destruction which clearly violates the divine dominion over human life.

On the other hand, the common consent of mankind clearly recognizes the fact that a man is not expected to sustain his life at all costs. The ultimate dissolution of the substance is likewise a part of nature.

These extremes are quite simple. It is in the vast area between that the real problems lie.

Review of Moral Opinions: These problems should become more clear as we inspect and attempt to evaluate the classical moral opinions on this subject, as well as the opinions of more recent theologians. Thereafter we shall try to formulate some working principles, drawn partially from both of these sources.

Classical Opinions:

St. Alphonsus Liguori sums up the moral opinion of the sixteenth and seventeenth centuries regarding this question, with a reference to the moral theology text of the Jesuit, Paul Laymann, that had appeared about a century before St. Alphonsus wrote, and was the popular seminary text.

Alphonsus quotes Laymann as teaching that no one is held to extraordinary and very difficult means to preserve his life, such as the amputation of a leg, unless his life be necessary for the common good. Alphonsus then adds that this is the common opinion to be found in the current moral treatises, and refers to the Jesuit DeLugo, the Dominicans Soto and Bannez, and to the secular priests, Tournely and Sylvius, together with the Salmanticenses of the Carmelites, as holding the same opinion.[19]

It is interesting to note here that while Saint Alphonsus speaks of "extraordinary and very difficult means; for example, the amputation of a leg," and refers to DeLugo, among others, as the source of his doctrine, DeLugo himself does not presuppose the extraordinary difficulty of a leg amputation, as Alphonsus seems to do. DeLugo says that a person "should permit that cure when the doctors indicate it as necessary, and when it can be done without intense pain." But he contradicts the amputation "if it would be accompanied by very intense pain, because no one is obliged to use extraordinary and very difficult means to preserve his life. . ."[20]

This is significant because a great deal of the difficulty in the question of ordinary and extraordinary means for the preservation of life seems to have stemmed from the apparent neglect of some of the moral theologians to give sufficient consideration to the advances in surgery and anesthesia. It would seem that DeLugo may have been thinking far ahead of his time.

For the same reason, it is interesting to note that Palmieri, writing a strictly Liguorian moral theology around 1830, retains the example of the leg amputation but adds: "if the pain is very great."[21]

The same caution is not characteristic of Bucceroni. In the 1914 edition of his work, we find the same common doctrine: the absence of any obligation to use what he calls, "exquisite remedies which cause great pain, for example, the amputation of a leg." And then apparently feeling that the amputation example is becoming a bit threadbare, having been in constant use since the sixteenth century, he adds another example of a remedy which causes great pain: "the incision of the abdomen to remove a stone."[22]

The medical world was aware of the fact that Augustus of Poland had sustained an amputation under total narcosis before 1872, and by 1900 the science of anesthesia was well on its way to perfection.

Yet the same brief answer, with the same threadbare examples, can be found in the 1925 edition of Ferreres' moral compendium,[23] and the 1928 edition of Colli-Lanzi's moral theology,[24] and when we find the same "amputation of a leg" and "incision of the abdomen to remove a stone" described in the

·same language in the 1944 edition of Aertnys-Damen,[25] the whole concept suggests an insufficient adaptation of the moral thinking to the current medical developments.

On the other hand, before 1898, Dr. Capellmann, who was also a moral theologian in his own right, reviewed the standard authors in his *Medicina Pastoralis* very much as we have done here, and observed that it was certainly of some moment that very difficult operations could then be performed without pain, thanks to chloroform, and that if one were to speak of the post-operative pains, "these generally are not so very difficult, and for the most part are less severe than those which the illness, which made the operation necessary, would bring on, and the sick man would have to bear these even without the operation."[26]

Even at this early date, Dr. Capellmann suggested that the theologians might do well to modify their opinions. He also pointed out that even in his day, the danger of major operations had been considerably lessened by the use of more efficient antiseptics.[27]

There were those, however, who were modifying the early Liguorian approach in view of the advances of medicine and surgery. The modifications which Capellmann suggested are found in the 1883 edition of Konings.[28] In the other cases the development was more gradual. Compare the following passages from the 1922, and then the 1941, editions of Noldin, the latter being Noldin's work, as revised by Schmitt.

Noldin (1922): "There is no obligation to undergo a serious surgical operation, or a notable amputation: even though today the pains of many operations are not acute, due to anesthetics, nevertheless, the obligation is not to be imposed, both because many have a great horror of it, and because the success, especially the lasting success, ordinarily is uncertain, and finally, because it is a grave inconvenience to live with a mutilated body."[29]

Noldin-Schmitt (1941): "Today the suffering is vastly decreased through narcotics, the danger of infection is very remote, and moreover success is more frequent and assured, and even for amputated members, there are artificial limbs—and therefore, at least where certain danger of death would very probably be avoided through an operation, it does not seem that it can be called an extraordinary means, unless there is great subjective horror of it."[30]

Finally, it is interesting to note that the very popular moral text (Jone-Adelman), regarding this matter in its first (1948) edition, reads, in part, as follows: "Neither is anyone gravely obliged to undergo a very dangerous operation. . ."[31]

More Recent Authors: In general the more recent authors followed the standard moralists in agreeing that man is obliged to take the ordinary means to preserve his life, but is not obliged to use extraordinary means, unless some element of the common good enters into the picture. All agreed that means which would involve extreme pain, danger of death, excessive expense, or great subjective repugnance were to be classified as extraordinary.

But all this was clearly delineated in the sixteenth century. When the real question arose, namely: are the advances of modern medicine in general to be classified as ordinary, or extraordinary means; and in particular, what is to be said of modern surgery, X-ray treatment, Wangensteen tubes, oxygen tents, iron lungs and intravenous feeding; they went riding madly off in all directions.

As medical progress advanced through the mid-twentieth century, there was a period of renewed theological speculation in an effort to identify various procedures as ordinary, or extraordinary. It will be helpful to discuss some of these here, since they pointed the direction of developing thought.

After repeating the standard principle on ordinary and extraordinary means, Lehmkuhl had strongly implied that ordinary means are to be identified with normal everyday eating, drinking, and sleeping.[32] We find this same implication in the Jone-Adelman text[33] and in *The Catholic Doctor* by Bonnar.[34] Moreover, Father Joseph McAllister, of the Catholic University of America, positively asserted the identity of ordinary means and natural means in his *Ethics*. Father McAllister's passage is quoted as a summary of this opinion regarding ordinary and extraordinary means of preserving life.

". . . a person is bound to use only the ordinary means of preserving his life. This includes proper diet and exercise and relaxation and sleep and all natural aids, which by its constitution the body needs to keep well. A surgical operation is not such a natural aid. It may not be against nature, but it certainly is not a provision of nature for man's welfare. In this sense it remains unnatural and extraordinary, and a person is not obliged to undergo it. . ."[35]

Artificial Not Wholly Distinct from Natural: We believe that the above opinion is untenable. It would seem to lead to a position wherein the modern antibiotics, by the mere fact that they are artificially produced and administered, would be considered extraordinary means of preserving life.

Moreover, although we must note and remember for future consideration that there is a valid distinction between natural and artificial means, still the artificial is not to be considered as wholly distinct from the natural.

The advances of modern science are due fundamentally to the development of the natural potentialities of civilized man living in society, with each generation building on the discoveries and achievements of the last, as is evidently in accord with the rational nature of man. Thus it is inauspicious to say that surgery, intravenous feeding, radiation therapy, and the like, are extraordinary means, because they are, in themselves, artificial and unnatural. They are not properly considered in themselves, but rather must be viewed in their historical context.

Just as the life of the individual advances and develops in complexity and perfection according to its natural potentialities, so, in the divine plan, a civilization or a culture develops. Thus what is extraordinary in one stage of cultural or scientific development, may be quite ordinary in another.

Ordinary Identified with Commonly Used: Another mid-century approach to the problem adhered to the lines of De-Lugo's 16th Disputation, where we find the ideas of "common" and "which men commonly use," juxtaposed with "ordinary."[36]

Thus, in somewhat the same vein, Healy, in his *Moral Guidance*, defined extraordinary as that which is "beyond the ordinary power of men," and while granting that an operation without anesthetic would be extraordinary, added that "today, however, anesthetics remove all such pain and so ordinarily (he) would be bound to have the operation."[37]

We believe that this is a much more tenable opinion, but that it leaves a still incomplete basis for judging what is an ordinary, and what is an extraordinary means of preserving life.

Investigation by an Example: To treat each advance of modern medicine in detail would require the dimensions of a book. As a fairly typical example we will consider the question of intravenous feeding. The conclusions will be applicable to many of the other modern medical and surgical advances and techniques.

Donovan, Sullivan, and Kelly classified intravenous feeding as an ordinary means of preserving life. The rudimentary case with which they dealt is described simply as that of a man dying, whose life can be prolonged for several weeks by intravenous injections.

Father Joseph Donovan wrote that in this case intravenous feeding must be considered an ordinary means, and that to stop it, would be equivalent to mercy killing.[38]

Both Father Gerald Kelly and Father Joseph Sullivan held that the means was, at least in itself, ordinary; but they likewise allowed circumstances wherein it could be licitly discontinued. In this way they added a further refinement of the principle.

Father Kelly, writing in *Theological Studies*, said: "I agree with Father Donovan that intravenous feeding is, in itself, an ordinary means. But even granted that it is ordinary, one may not immediately conclude that it is obligatory. . . To me, the mere prolonging of life in the given circumstances seems to be relatively useless, and I see no sound reason for saying that the patient is obliged to submit to it."[39]

Father Joseph Sullivan, in his *Catholic Teaching on the Morality of Euthanasia*, while likewise allowing that intravenous feeding is an ordinary means in itself, added to the case the circumstance of great pain which could be alleviated only briefly due to drug toleration, and said that intravenous feeding is, however, an artificial means, and that in such a case it could be considered extraordinary and be discontinued.[40]

It is extremely important to notice that both Father Kelly and Father Sullivan considered intravenous feeding, in itself, to be an ordinary means of prolonging life, yet in certain cases both sanctioned its discontinuance: Father Kelly, because "the mere prolonging of life in the given circumstances seems to be relatively useless," and Father Sullivan, because "an artificial means of preserving life may be an ordinary means or an extraordinary means relative to the physical condition of the patient."

Proposed Solution: In the quotations just cited from Father Kelly and Father Sullivan it appears that each of them had pried a little more deeply into the basic principle than anyone else since DeLugo's time. Each of them gave reasons why means which are ordinary in themselves may be discontinued under certain circumstances. While their reasons appear to be different, the word "relative" is the key word in each quotation. Perhaps the word "relative" is the key word in the whole problem.

Let us begin with the notion of "absolutes" and "relatives" in the context of man's strivings. We speak of ends which absolutely must be achieved, at any cost; we might define such an end as a good that is so essential to the very nature of man that it is either the ultimate end itself, or so necessary a means to that ultimate end that no effort or cost could be conceived which would be proportionate to the loss of such good. Examples would be beatitude, or supernatural charity.

But the very concept of a *"finis absolute obtinendus"* postulates the concept of a *"finis relative obtinendus."* This, in turn, we might define as a good which, according to right order, must be sought with that amount of effort and cost that is reckoned to be in proportion with the actual contribution of the good, once obtained, to the totality of man's nature and the pursuit of his ultimate end.

No one would classify the prolongation of human life, in itself, such an "absolute." It is, in itself, a relative value. And granting that the prolongation of human life is a good which is to be obtained relatively, our question is precisely this: relatively to what?

To answer this question we must ask another. What, precisely, is the meaning of human life, as such, in the present cosmic dispensation of divine Providence? In other words, why, ultimately, must human life be preserved?

We have already seen that man should not positively and voluntarily terminate his life span. But, moreover, man must preserve his life because it is the fundamental natural and God-given good, the fundamental context in which all the other goods must be exercised.

Therefore the meaning of "relativity" in the preservation of life seems to be the relation of a due proportion between the cost and effort required to preserve this fundamental context, and the potentialities of the other goods that still remain to be worked out within that context.

If we now formulate a definition of ordinary means from the opinions and arguments just reviewed, and take this definition as a common denominator for working out cases on this formula of relativity, we should have what we set out to find, that is, the grounds for a reasonable moral judgment in most cases. It is to be noted that what we are looking for here is not a new definition of ordinary means, but rather a definition drawn from the critical evaluation of the standard authors. Using this definition in conjunction with what we hope is a clearer delineation of the relativity involved, we must not expect to find a "moral slide rule," which will automatically answer cases, but rather the ultimate grounds for the necessary moral judgment. It must be noted here that this approach does not reduce the question to a "situation ethic." The determining factors of morality include moral object, motive and circumstances. The absolutes remain intact in the exclusion of positive euthanasia and suicide as "moral objects." The "situation" enters only into the evaluation of the circumstances with such considerations as, in a given case, when does therapy cease to be therapeutic?

Summary of Conclusions:

1. Ordinary means might best be defined as those which are at hand, and do not entail effort, suffering, or expense beyond that which men would consider proper for a serious undertaking, according to the state of life of each individual and the financial resources (insurance, etc.) available.

2. Apart from subjective considerations of pain, expense, or personal abhorrence (which classic authors generally used as a partial basis for judging means to be extraordinary), most of the commonly available techniques of modern surgery and medicine should be classified as ordinary means of preserving life.

3. The use of these developed techniques, as ordinary means, is to be distinguished from the every day actions of eating, drinking, and sleeping.

4. These developed techniques need not be used in some circumstances. The relation of their use to the remaining potentiality of what we have called "the fundamental context of human life," should be the basis of the moral judgment as to whether such modern means must be used or not. In those cases where an obligation to use such means cannot be demonstrated, the means might be considered as "relatively extraordinary."

A Word of Caution: One further consideration should be added in the form of a caution. We must not be too ready to terminate the use of either ordinary or extraordinary means of prolonging life, even though, in itself, such termination would be morally justified in a given case. This for three reasons:

First, there is the danger that such an attitude could be construed in the minds of some as a sort of "Catholic euthanasia." It is the same caution, for the same reason, that advises prudence in the treating of periodic continence, lest the charge of "Catholic birth control" be incurred in a misinterpreted sense.

Secondly, there is in the medical profession an ideal which demands the fighting off of pain and death until the last possible moment. It is safe to say that many of the great advances in modern medicine, as well as a perfection and skill in technique, have been due to what might frequently have been called a "useless prolonging of life." If, for example, modern surgery is an ordinary means of preserving life, it is only so because of its extensive use in those stages of its development when it was an extraordinary means. This consideration bears directly upon the common good. Father Kelly warned against a defeatist attitude, which would "turn back the clock" of medical progress, and we must not be too ready to risk a lowering of the medical ideal, and a retardation of medical progress in the immediate interests of the individual case.

Thirdly, it must be kept in mind that the doctor is acting as the agent of the patient, or of the next of kin. Therefore, the wishes of these are to be respected. If the patient or the next of kin want extraordinary means to be continued, or to be discontinued, it is the doctor's duty to respect their wishes.

This third point needs immediate further consideration: who is to make the decision to discontinue relatively extraordinary means in the concrete circumstances of a given case?

The question of decision by next of kin or physician arises only when the patient is unable to decide, an inability that may be due to unconsciousness or even extreme emotional instability. At this point, if a decision is to be made, it must be made vicariously, but it is being made for the patient and must follow the interpreted desires of the patient in the context of the reasonable alternatives.

Several suppositions have traditionally left this determination to the next of kin (or some individuals of the immediate family). First, there is the supposition that such are most likely to be able to best interpret what the patient would wish. This supposition may, indeed, yield to contrary fact, and in the context of family practice, it may be the family physician who will have the better insight here.

Second, there is the supposition that the next of kin will be paying the bills, and this consideration relates to the "reasonable alternatives" just mentioned. There are certainly cases in which the next of kin could not reasonably be expected to purchase extraordinary medical services that would be neither morally obligatory nor that he would be inclined to purchase even for himself.

Third, there is the supposition (and consideration) of the inextricability of the next of kin's familial relationship in a situation demanding decision. The physician can, after all, arrange to withdraw from the case in the presence of decisions offending either his medical ideal, or his moral sense, but the family of the patient cannot withdraw from familial responsibility.

Finally, it could be that sometimes there is an unfortunate iatrogenic aura of proprietorship over the patient that is due more to popular idiom than to idea, but that might conflict with what others view as a more humane mind. When the physician says "my patient," he only overtones his desire to do his very best for the sick, but where there are valid options, his medical idea of "best," might generate an understandable caution in the public course. By such a course, I obviously do not mean killing, compassionate or otherwise, but rather the sympathetic desire to let the patient die in peace.

It is the physician who will be more familiar with most of the reasonable alternatives (since they will be mostly medical), and better able to judge the cost of continued extraordinary measures, and better able to assess the anticipated emotional drain on the family as the final illness is slowed down to what may be, for them, a tortured approach to finality.

Terminal illness often demands a decision, becoming one of those exigent human situations in which even not to make a decision is, in itself, to decide. What is important is the recognition that the right to decide belongs radically to the patient. If circumstances demand that a decision must be made for him, then it must be accurately vicarious insofar as it can be. This is what requires an estimate of the patient's wishes in the context of the available alternatives. In the moral frame, there has been a general supposition that someone in the relationship of next of kin can best interpret the wishes, not because of some consanguineous prerogative, but because of more intimate knowledge of the patient. That supposition may yield to contrary fact, and at times (and here I prescind from possible legal complications and restrict myself to the moral considerations), the appropriate awareness of what the patient would wish may reside with a friend or other close associate, or not infrequently with the family physician. Thus the family, and the physician, and perhaps also some other intimate of the patient might best approach the decision together, knowing that they are vicegerents seeking to decide according to the interpreted wishes of the patient, and not on their own.

Conscientious Objections to Therapy

The most perplexing problems of prolongation of life in terminal illness arise in those cases in which the rights and freedom of conscience of the individual patient, the ideals and freedom of conscience of the individual physician, and sometimes the prerogatives of the State seem to all meet and clash. Perhaps the most typical and recurrent of these situations involves the Jehovah's Witness[41] and the question of blood transfusion. The moral analysis of other similar conscientious objections to a particular therapy would be essentially the same.

Although blood transfusion is not without some danger of serious side effects, most people today consider it to be an ordinary life-saving procedure. The authentic Jehovah's Witness, however, refuses blood transfusion as a tenet of religious conviction. The case is liable to assume one of three aspects.

First is the case of the adult patient who is seriously ill and in grave need of the transfusion. Whether the patient is conscious and refuses permission for the transfusion or is unconscious but has previously refused the transfusion on religious grounds, the situation is essentially the same. It is a violation of human rights either to give the transfusion or to seek a court order whereby the transfusion would be effected. In some cases such court orders have been granted, in other cases they have been denied.

This is the easiest of the three cases, and the reasons for the opinion presented here are as follows. While one is obliged to use ordinary means to prolong his life, one is not obliged to use extraordinary means. Theologians agree that what is, in itself, an ordinary means can be considered *subjectively extraordinary* if the patient has a grave subjective abhorrence, antipathy, repugnance or aversion to its use. This is a subjective state of mind on the part of the patient which *de facto* can exist whether the considerations which give rise to it are reasonable or not. This is certainly verified in the Jehovah's Witness with regard to transfusion. Since, therefore, the transfusion is properly considered to be a subjectively extraordinary means of prolonging the life of this patient, the patient has no obligation to resort to it. Hence, the patient has a right to refuse it, and no matter what the consequences to the patient may be, that right must be respected.

The second case is more difficult. What is to be done if the patient is an infant in need of transfusion as a life-saving therapy, and the parents or the next of kin refuse permission?

In this case the more usual disposition of the courts has been to declare the child a ward of the State and to order the transfusion. The situation is usually approached under the juvenile court law of the various jurisdictions which provides, in some degree, for the protection of "dependent and neglected children." The procedure is ultimately based on the common law concept of the State as *parens patriae.*

This is a morally sound approach to the problem. It is true that the State must recognize the right of the individual to freedom of conscience. But while freedom of conscience insures the right to believe what one believes, it does not insure the right to act on that belief in every aspect of human relationships, particularly when to do so would be in violation of the rights of others. In this apparent conflict the State is correct in assuming the custody of the child to insure that the child receives ordinary care. Moreover, it should be noted that the transfusion remains an ordinary means for preserving the infant life, since the child does not experience that personal abhorrence which made the transfusion subjectively extraordinary in the previous case.

Other legal complications which might arise in this case, such as the restricted right of the physician to testify in the court process regarding privileged communications or the right of the parents to trial by jury, are legal rather than moral problems. From a moral viewpoint, such lesser rights would yield to the higher right of the child to life, and the legal approach would be a matter for the court to decide.

The third and most difficult case is that of the mother who is in need of life-saving transfusion, and is carrying her unborn child in her womb.

Such a case came before the Supreme Court of the State of New Jersey on June 17, 1964 in regard to a patient at Fitkin Memorial Hospital. The court recognized the fact that the pregnancy was beyond the thirty-second week, and that the mother was in danger of hemorrhage which would be fatal to both herself and the unborn child. After the Chancery Division of the Superior Court held that the judiciary could not intervene, the Supreme Court did not hesitate to order the transfusion for the protection of the unborn child.[42]

Here we have the unusual situation of the court being right in principle, but perhaps wrong in this particular application of the principle. Theologians would certainly agree with the court's insistence on the right of the unborn child to the protection of the law. Moreover it is interesting to note that in the twenty years prior to the Supreme Court's more recent death-dealing decisions in regard to unborn babies,[43] there had been a healthy legal trend away from the view established by a decision of Justice Holmes in 1884, refusing to recognize the legal existence of an unborn child.

The mother certainly has an objective obligation to provide ordinary care for her unborn child, and if she refuses to do this, for whatever reason, the State, as *parens patriae*, has a right to step in. However, under the peculiar circumstances of this kind of case, perhaps the State should not exercise that right; even if both the mother and the child will otherwise die—and this for two reasons.

First, to force a conscious Jehovah's Witness, on the point of death, to submit to a blood transfusion to save the life of her unborn child, might well bring her human and religious feelings into such deep and confusing conflict, as to endanger her own spiritual welfare at this uncertain and critical moment. Hence, even if the obligation for her to accept the transfusion is verified, it should not be urged under these circumstances at the risk of her eternal salvation.

Secondly, the precedent of the State physically invading the human person contrary to her conscience is so dangerous to the common good as to outweigh the individual good of the unborn child.

One other recent development in the general problem of the Jehovah's Witness and the blood transfusion should be noted. Although there has been some discussion as to whether or not blood collected in advance from, and reserved for the use of, a particular patient could be acceptable to a Jehovah's Witness for autotransfusion, this proposed solution has been rejected by *The Watchtower Bible and Tract Society* (New York) which is an official organ of the Jehovah's Witnesses.[44]

Artificial Resuscitation

The literature on the problem of artificial resuscitation, particularly after cardiac arrest, reflects a growing tendency among many physicians to question the propriety of continued efforts for resuscitation in the presence of severe brain damage due to anoxia. And even aside from these cases, some suggest that prior to dramatic efforts at artificial resuscitation at any time, one should question whether the patient has the fundamental health to justify the procedure. Hamilton Southworth wrote, in this regard: "Obviously one would not resuscitate a patient with terminal carcinoma or an overwhelming myocardial infarct."[45] On somewhat the same vein, Father John Connery, S.J., writes that, from a moral viewpoint, cardiac massage after extensive brain damage would undoubtedly be considered an extraordinary means of prolonging life and concludes: "While a doctor should certainly comply with the wishes of relatives if they request it immediately after apparent death, I think the physician should advise against any such measures after the 3-5 minutes has elapsed."[46]

Father Connery is using the "3-5 minutes" measure as a current norm in ordinary circumstances as reported in the medical literature. The details of time limits and the extent of cerebral deterioration, whether arising from prenatal asphyxia, neonatal obstructions, erythroblastosis, or some perinatal accident; or, in the adult, from drowning, aspiration of the stomach contents, poliomyelitis, poisoning, brain surgery, anesthetic catastrophe or any other cause, are the proper subjects of medical investigation. Haldane coined a phrase in the early 1920's which has become axiomatic when he pointed out that this type of insult "not only stops the machine, but wrecks the machinery." He likewise presented the fourfold classification of anoxia, depending upon the proximate cause of oxygen deficiency, as stagnant anoxia (due to a circulatory defect inhibiting the flow of the fuel-bearing blood), anemic anoxia (a deficiency of the amount of oxygen-bearing hemoglobin in the blood stream), anoxic anoxia (due to a limitation at the supply center, the alveoli of the lungs), or finally histiotoxic anoxia (due to tissue damage at the point of delivery inhibiting uptake).

When one or more of these processes results in inadequate oxygenation of the tissues of the brain and central nervous system, the results in these highly susceptible nerve cells are serious. The effects may vary in different areas and will vary with different types of anoxia. In general, acute cases are said to result in congestion and focal hemorrhages of the brain, followed by progressive degeneration of the cells of the cerebral cortex and basic ganglia and progressively through other areas. Courville's earlier observation regarding this process pinpoints the moral problem: "Once set in motion by the acute anoxia process, the structural alterations in the brain are usually progressive in nature up to a given point. . . There is clinical evidence that would indicate that changes in the nerve cells at least are reversible to a considerable degree if the original insult is not too profound."[47]

The moral question, then, comes down to this: What obligation is there to continue artificial means of resuscitation and support of vital functions, when sound medical judgment indicates that extensive and irreversible brain damage has already taken place, or when the patient's general condition implies a negative prognosis due to extensive and debilitating disease?

Bearing in mind the previous considerations on prolongation of life in terminal illness, it may safely be said that when a patient has suffered brain damage to such an extent that survival will not include the ability to lead a life even approximating the normal; or when, even apart from such damage due to anoxia, disease processes have debilitated the patient beyond any hopeful prognosis, it is very likely that a consideration of all the circumstances of the individual case will lead to the sound moral judgment that artificial resuscitation, whether manual or mechanical, may be considered in that particular case to be a relatively extraordinary means of prolonging life.

Once this judgment is reached, then the wishes of the patient (either previously made known or presently interpreted), become the operative norm for further treatment. In this regard Pope Pius XII pointed out that: "The rights and duties of the family depend on the presumed will of the unconscious patient, if he is of age and *sui juris*. Where the proper and independent duty of the family is concerned, they are usually bound to use only ordinary means."[48]

This decision can become more burdensome, because, in the context of modern emergency medicine, mechanical respirators and resuscitators are often in operation before any other considerations are made, and the question of shutting them off gives rise to far more anxiety and moral tension than an earlier decision not to employ them in a particular case would have done. Pius XII clearly had this case in mind also when, referring to such measures as extraordinary in some circumstances, he urged that the Anointing of the Sick be administered to the Catholic patient before resuscitation is stopped, and also pointed out that even when such discontinuance caused circulatory arrest, it was not, for that reason, morally wrong or in any way comparable to euthanasia.[49]

CHAPTER FOUR

MORAL ASPECTS OF SURGERY AND SUPPRESSIVE THERAPY

We have seen that the proper concepts of right order in human life properly ascribe to man an administrative role of stewardship with regard to the gift of life which he has received.

In the course of professional practice, the doctor, acting as the agent of his patient, will be called upon to undertake procedures which result in a positive invasion of the body's functional integrity. Indications are recognized which call for the removal of some organ or the suppression of its function in the interest of the whole body.

Briefly, if the procedure is strictly an act of wise administration and the proper exercise of stewardship, it is morally right; but if it is an act of ownership and a usurpation of God's absolute prerogative, and in violation of the immanent teleology of the body and its parts, it is morally wrong.

"Mutilation" as a Technical Term: The use of the word *mutilation* as it occurs in theological writings calls for a brief explanation. The word is found as a technical term with a meaning not quite the same as that associated with its ordinary usage. It is derived from the Latin: *mutilare,* which is used in classical literature by both Livy and Ovid in the familiar sense of: *to maim or distort,* and the latter also uses it simply to mean: *amputate.* Cicero uses the same word to mean: *diminish or lessen.* The English derivative: mutilation, entered the clinical vocabulary with a more specific meaning and is defined by Dorland's Medical Dictionary as: "the act of depriving a limb, member or important part; deprival of an organ." And the medical-moral

definition is simply: "the removal of an organ or the suppression of its function."

As will be explained more fully in the subsequent pages, when discussing the morality of surgical removal or pharmacological suppression, one must immediately distinguish between those procedures which do, or do not affect the generative function. Outside the generative system, such procedures are governed by the principle of totality, whereas within the generative system one must also have recourse to the principle of double effect.

The Principle of Totality

An abstract expression of the principle of totality is merely the fact that the parts of a physical entity, as parts, are ordained to the good of the physical whole. Since this good of the whole is the fundamental meaning of, and reason for, the existence of the parts, there is no violation of right order in the destruction of the parts, when this is necessary for the good of the whole.

Concretely, the principle of totality means that all the parts of the human body, as parts, are meant to exist and function for the good of the whole body, and are thus naturally subordinated to the good of the whole body.

Therefore, when some part or function becomes detrimental to the good of the whole body, as for example an infected appendix, a gangrenous leg, or a malfunctioning spleen, it is in accord with right order to remove such a part or to suppress its function.

It is to be noted that in such cases there is no need of invoking the principle of double effect. The procedure may result in some physical evil, such as the loss of a leg, but there is no question of "moral evil" and hence no "evil effect" in the technical sense of that term. The justifiable mutilation is directly intended. The teleology of generative organs goes beyond this relationship of part to whole, and so, questions involving them will be given consideration subsequently in these pages.

The principle of totality has been expressed by Pius XII as follows:

Considered as a whole, the physical organism of living beings, of plants, animals, or man has a unity subsisting in itself. Each of the members, for example, the hand, the foot, the heart, the eye, is an integral part destined by all its being to be inserted into the whole organism. Outside the organism it has not, by its very nature, any sense, any finality . . .

What results as far as the physical organism is concerned? The master and user of this organism, which possesses a subsisting unity, can dispose directly and immediately of the integral parts, members, and organs, within the scope of their natural finality. He can also intervene, as often as, and to the extent that, the good of the whole demands, to paralyze, destroy, mutilate, and separate the members.[50]

While the principle of totality thus permits impairment for the good of the whole body, on the other hand man's *merely useful* prerogative over his body likewise limits justified mutilation and restricts it to those situations wherein it is necessary for the good of the whole body.

This limitation was expressed clearly by Pius XI in his encyclical letter on Christian marriage, as follows:

Furthermore, Christian doctrine establishes, and the light of human reason makes it most clear, that private individuals have no other power over the members of their own bodies than that which pertains to their natural ends: and they are not free to destroy or mutilate their members, or in any other way render themselves unfit for their natural functions, except when no other provision can be made for the good of the whole body.[51]

Procedures within the Generative System

Just as clearly as the various parts of the body mentioned above, such as the heart, lungs, liver, spleen, etc., bear a very definite relation to the good of the whole body, so likewise the generative organs bear this same relation of part to whole. But, *in addition to this*, the generative organs also bear a very definite relationship transcending the good of the individual.

Thus, although a generative organ is physically one, it must be considered under two distinct aspects, because of its twofold diversity of function and purpose.

First, as parts of the body, the testes, ovaries, tubes, ducts, etc., exist for the good of the whole body, just as the arms, legs, heart, liver, spleen, etc. If, precisely as parts, they are destructive of the good of the whole body, they may be removed or functionally suppressed.

These organs of generation have, however, another function and meaning as "parts"; namely, their function and meaning as "generative." Moreover, precisely "as generative" they do not exist only for the good of the individual, but their teleology extends beyond the individual and relates directly not only to the good of the species, but also to the deeply inter-personal integrity of that unique communication of oblative love which is the marriage act.

Therefore, according to right order, precisely in so far as they are generative their significance is not solely the good of the individual.

To clarify and retain this distinction for future reference, let us note clearly what we mean by a "therapeutic procedure" as opposed to a "contraceptive procedure" within the generative system.

A Therapeutic Procedure: A procedure is said to be therapeutic when a generative organ is removed or its function is suppressed in so far as the organ, precisely as part of the body, is destructive of the good of the whole body. An example of this would be the removal of a cancerous uterus.

A Contraceptive Procedure: A procedure is said to be contraceptive when a generative organ is removed or its function is suppressed in so far as the organ is a medium of generation, and for the purpose of destroying its generative function. An example of this would be sterilization in the presence of some cardiac disease.

In accord with these considerations, the Catholic Church teaches that a therapeutic procedure, directly intended as therapeutic, is permitted, but a directly intended contraceptive procedure is wrong, precisely because the latter is beyond the scope of man's prerogative in regard to his own body. A more detailed treatment of the Catholic teaching on contraception will be found in the chapter on marriage. It is sufficient to note here that since many procedures in the generative system actually will necessarily be both therapeutic and contraceptive *in result*, the principle of the double effect must be employed. In such procedures the good effect, directly intended, will be the therapeutic result; while the evil effect, not intended but foreseen and merely permitted, will be the contraceptive result. But again it should be clearly understood that when a contraceptive result is intended as a means to a therapeutic end (as in sterilization to prevent pregnancy in the presence of cardiac or renal disease), the sterilization is called "direct" or "directly contraceptive" and is contrary to Catholic teaching.

Suppression or Excision of a Healthy Organ

Some writers, due possibly to a misinterpretation of Saint Thomas's treatment of mutilation,[52] have demanded that an organ be diseased before its removal is justified. This is incorrect. It is a distinction not even mentioned by many of the standard moral theologians, expressly denied by others, and is clearly incompatible with the following statement of Pope Pius XII in his address to the Twenty-sixth Annual Convention of the Italian Society of Urologists:

> The decisive point here is not that the organ that is removed or rendered functionless is itself diseased, but that its preservation or its function entails either directly or indirectly a serious threat to the whole body. It is quite possible that by its normal functioning a healthy organ may exercise an influence of such a nature on a diseased organ as to aggravate the disease and its consequences throughout the whole body. It can also happen that the removal of a healthy organ and the suppression of its normal functioning will remove from a disease, cancer, for example, its field of growth, or, in any case, essentially change the conditions of its existence. If there is no other means at our disposal,

surgical intervention on the healthy organ is permitted in both cases.

The conclusion that we have reached is deduced from the right of disposition that man has received from the Creator in regard to his own body, in accord with the principle of totality, which is valid here also, and in virtue of which each particular organ is subordinated to the whole body and must yield to it in case of conflict....[53]

But it is to be noted (as indicated above) in the same address the Roman Pontiff explicitly added that the same principle of totality could not be rightly used to defend a directly contraceptive sterilization, even in order to preclude a pregnancy which might complicate some other present condition, such as cardiac or kidney disease, for example.

Blood Transfusion and Skin Grafting

Regarding those procedures wherein a part of the skin is removed for purposes of grafting, even to another person; or a quantity of blood is removed for transfusion; these are not mutilations in the theological sense of the word because these parts are quickly restored, and the integrity of the body is not lessened to any notable degree.

The fact that some members of the normal human body exist in duplicate, such as the upper and lower extremities, eyes, ears, and generative glands, etc., does not justify the unwarranted removal of only one of them, because thereafter the body is no longer functionally integral.

In fetal anomalies, like polydactylism, the removal of the extra digit or other parts cannot be called mutilation, since such removal would be for the correction of an anomaly. Such a procedure would result in a contribution to, rather than a lessening of, the physical integrity.

As explained in the pages immediately preceding, there is no serious moral problem involved in the surgical removal of a diseased appendix, gall bladder, spleen, kidney, lung, etc. It is possible, however, to envision a difficulty in this matter in the light of the already quoted words of Pius XI: "They are not free to destroy or mutilate their members . . . except when no other provision can be made for the good of the whole body."

Obviously the words: "no other provision" are to be taken in a reasonable sense and in context with "good of the whole body." They should not be understood to mean that mutilation is never permissible when there is any other available way of preserving life. If such were the case, a man with gall bladder disease, for example, faced with the alternatives of surgical intervention or long, expensive, and discomforting treatment, would be obliged to forego the surgery in favor of the treatment. This is clearly not true.

Father Francis Connell, C.SS.R., considerably clarified this concept in the following words:

> According to Catholic moral principles, the mutilation or excision of a part of the body is permitted only when there is certainty or probability that benefit will thereby come to the whole body in sufficient measure to compensate for the harm that has been done.[55]

Moreover, it is to be remembered that just as the parts, precisely as parts, are subordinated to the good of the whole body; so likewise the body itself, as a part, is subordinated to the good of the whole person. And although procedures less drastic than surgery might be able to preserve the existence or "being" of the body, they may not be as contributory as surgery, in many instances, to the "well-being" either of the body or of the whole person.

Cosmetic Surgery

Sometimes questions arise with regard to surgery, whether major or minor, which is done for purposes of improving the appearance of the body. Anomalies or malfunctions of the body, either congenital or induced by trauma, can be a definite psychological and even financial handicap. Many such cases represent aberrations from the normal and, moreover, the appearance of the individual does have an impact upon his adaptation to society. Hence cosmetic surgery is in accord with the principle of totality as long as there is a due proportion between the risk involved and the expected good. Nasal and auricular reconstructions, and the removal of moles and blemishes, are obvious examples of plastic surgery for cosmetic purposes.

Surgery for Prosthetic Substitution: Questions sometimes arise regarding amputation of a partially impaired member in order that a prosthesis may be substituted.

The congenitally atrophic upper extremity can usually be fitted with a prosthesis with little or no surgical interference, but a more complicated problem arises in hemiparesis, or partial paralysis limited to an otherwise normal arm, resulting in poor coordination of motion and very limited dexterity. Sometimes these individuals request the removal of the afflicted member and substitution of a prosthesis. If, after consultation, the surgeon and psychiatrist agree that such substitution would result in greater functional integrity, the procedure would not be morally contraindicated.

Unnecessary Surgery

In the light of the general principles already discussed, it seems unnecessary to add anything regarding the evident moral turpitude of unnecessary surgery in the sense of operations for which there is no real medical indication, but which might be undertaken for some unworthy motive such as financial gain or face-saving.

We hope that such practices are so rare as to scarcely merit comment. Moreover, Father Gerald Kelly, S.J., made the following particularly important and significant observation on this subject:

> It may be somewhat easy now to go back over the records and decide that some kind of surgery was unnecessary, but perhaps it was not so easy to make that judgment at the time the surgery was performed.[56]

Dr. Bernard J. Ficarra brings up another aspect of this concept in his book: *Newer Ethical Problems in Medicine and*

Surgery. Dr. Ficarra envisions the case of a surgeon who might be tempted to do a more radical procedure which is easier and less complicated rather than take the time and care, as well as the responsibility, of a more conservative operation even when the more conservative operation would be to the patient's greater benefit. Dr. Ficarra's point, which is well taken and worthy of serious consideration, is as follows:

> Culpability for mutilation may fall upon a surgeon in certain specific instances. For example, if a surgeon is called upon to treat a serious injury of the hand, forearm, arm, or leg and if the injury is of such severity that it is beyond his ability or knowledge to preserve or repair that injury, and if the surgeon amputates such an extremity rather than to ask for assistance, he has committed a moral tort. . .

> In another situation a surgeon may have occasion to treat a severe hand injury with extensive damage to tendons and adjacent structures. If there is a possibility that extensive surgical repair may preserve part or all of the hand, the surgeon is bound in conscience to do all in his power to preserve as much of the hand as possible. Although it would be easier for the surgeon to amputate, he is bound in the name of moral justice to conserve as much tissue as possible.[57]

Incidental Appendectomy

The questions of incidental and strictly elective appendectomy are taken up here in some detail partly to illustrate a structure of theological thinking which has unfortunately been neglected. In the more recent atmosphere as a vague sort of "Catholic Situationalism" there has been a tendency to substitute a sort of "holistic" intuition for careful analysis, but the parameters of right order are more properly approached in the context of right reason.

During the course of general abdominal surgery a healthy appendix is sometimes removed as a precautionary measure against some future danger. It is safe to say that today most surgeons look upon this procedure as sound prophylaxis, provided it does not involve any additional danger. With the same

precautionary provision there is no moral objection to this practice; presupposing, of course, the consent of the patient.

As far as determinable to date, the adult vermiform appendix
is a functionless organ which very definitely constitutes a potential danger, even if it is not diseased at the moment. Since the
patient is already under general anesthetic and the abdomen
is already open, the additional surgery involved in an incidental
appendectomy is so slight that any reasonable cause would justify
it. The removal of the danger of a later illness which would
require emergency surgery would justify it as a reasonable act
of wise administration, provided little or no risk is involved in
the additional surgical procedure. The added risk of infection
is, indeed, statistically minimal and the study of several cases has
shown that the appendix had already undergone occult and
undesirable pathologic changes in as high as 50% of the cases
reviewed.

This refinement of the principles regarding mutilation was
well delineated by Father Kelly:

> Since mutilations vary in degree, the reasons justifying
> them must also vary. The cure of a slight danger may justify
> a slight mutilation, whereas, the removal of an important part
> or the suppression of an important function requires a very
> serious reason. In other words, mutilations are justifiable for
> proportionate reasons that concern the preservation or res-
> toration of health.[58]

Strictly Elective Appendectomy

By strictly elective appendectomy we mean the removal of
a healthy appendix, not as described above, i.e., under circumstances in which the abdomen is already open for some other
reason; but as performed on a healthy individual and including
abdominal incision for the specific purpose of removing a healthy
appendix.

We do not believe that this prophylaxis against the possible
danger of a future appendicitis is in proportion to the risk of
abdominal surgery with its possibilities of untoward anesthetic
reactions and post-operative complications. Although modern
techniques and antibiotics have greatly reduced these risks, by

the same means the danger inherent in a future appendicitis is likewise reduced.

This is not meant to deny that there could be possible exceptions to this restriction. Such might be had, for example, in the case of an individual about to embark on a way of life wherein surgical attention would not be available in the future, as would actually be the case on some foreign missions. Under such circumstances, the statistical probability of a future serious appendicitis would seem to warrant such a precautionary measure, and we believe that such a strictly elective appendectomy would be morally permissible.

Danger is, after all, concerned with the probability of a future evil and since, in the case described above, the present moment is the ultimate opportunity for effective precaution, the danger might be said to be "relatively imminent."

Elective Tonsillectomy

The reasoning that is applied to incidental appendectomy does not apply to elective tonsillectomy. In the first place, the function of the tonsil is well known and the normal functioning of healthy tonsils does make a contribution to the physical well-being of the body. Moreover, the latent danger verified in the case of the appendix is not realized in regard to the tonsils and any danger involved in tonsillitis can be adequately counteracted by treatment and/or tonsillectomy after the organ has become affected.

Circumcision of the Newborn

Circumcision or the surgical removal of the distal part of the prepuce of the glans penis is obviously a justified surgical procedure when redundant foreskin interferes with micturation. Moralists, however, have questioned the routine practice of circumcision of the newborn when this is done irrespective of a clearly identified need. At least two authors have rejected routine circumcision without definite medical indication as morally objectionable. Father Gerald Kelly, S.J., on the other hand, expressed his opinion as follows:

Not a few doctors, however, consider that routine circumcision is advisable unless there are contrary indications. Since the mutilation is slight (in fact, many moralists would not designate it as a mutilation), I believe that our hospitals are justified in adopting a tolerant attitude toward these doctors. By this I mean that we need not oppose the procedure, as long as it is limited to cases in which circumcision is not actually contraindicated.

Father Kelly's opinion is adopted here with the following observations regarding parental consent, which must always be obtained.

1. In the case of the newborn, many parents will either reject circumcision or request it. Their wishes should be followed.

2. Other parents, when consulted, will leave the matter to the good judgment of the physician. In these latter cases the physician is perfectly free to advise circumcision if he feels that it is medically advantageous and not dangerous because of prematurity, blood abnormality, or some other contraindicative condition of the infant.

3. We have said "medically advantageous" instead of "medically necessary," because in cases where the mutilation is so slight and the surgical danger so remote we may properly speak of "advantages" rather than "necessity" in judging the licity of the procedure.

Dr. Richard Amelar lists some of these advantages: The occurrence of carcinoma of the penis in an individual circumcised at birth is so exceedingly rare that isolated case reports are widely quoted in the literature. It is generally agreed that complete prophylaxis against carcinoma is conferred by a well performed circumcision early in infancy. This fact, plus the ease of maintaining personal hygiene once the prepuce has been removed, accounts for the large number of circumcisions being performed today in this country on newborn males of all races and religions.[59]

There is another consideration which, if substantiated medically, would have significance in evaluating the morality of this surgical procedure. There is, on the part of some, strong suspicion corroborated by some evidence that the smegma which collects under the male prepuce not only constitutes a health hazard for the male but is likewise a carcinogenic agent in regard to the cervix of his spouse. At the present time this hypothesis is far too controversial to be of any real moral significance. Indeed, there are those physicians who energetically condemn routine circumcision of the newborn, and contend that the various medical reasons proposed to defend the practice are invalid. The weight of published medical opinion is, however, more favorable toward circumcision.[60]

Ghost Surgery

Ghost surgery is defined by the American College of Surgeons as surgery in which the patient is not informed of, or is misled, as to the identity of the operating surgeon.

It is a practice which the profession has publicly condemned, and this alone indicates that the evil is not just some theoretical possibility, but is a present reality in some quarters.

It is particularly interesting to note that the Judicial Council of the American Medical Association has condemned "ghost surgery," not only as unacceptable professional procedure, but in terms of a moral evil as an insult to the dignity of a human being, and in violation of the human rights of one's fellow man.[61]

Aside from the fact that the patient has an evident right to know and select the surgeon to whom he is to entrust his life, the moral evil here is mainly in the attendant injustice which is extremely likely to befall the patient.

If the referring surgeon is paid a surgical fee, it is money to which he has no right in justice. It is likely to matter very little to the patient if this form of injustice is avoided by the "ghost" surgeon's making a voluntary "kickback" to the referring surgeon, since in either case, it is extremely likely that it will be eventually the patient who pays.

Moreover, in such an arrangement, the operating surgeon is

likely to be excluded from the pre-operative examination and the post-operative care, and this is very likely to be detrimental to the patient's welfare.

Finally, even if the injustices mentioned above were to be avoided in particular cases, it is a practice which seriously militates against the common good, because it brings into disrepute a profession whose honor and esteem are necessary for the welfare of the community.

Residency Training Surgery

Residence training programs current in the United States today represent an adaptation from the German system in providing, as an integral part of the educational process, gradually increasing experience and responsibility in patient treatment and care.

Moral theologians and physicians alike have raised questions as to the ethical propriety of those aspects of such training programs which seem, in effect, very much like a thinly veiled form of "ghost surgery," as, for example, if the resident trainee, under the direction of the surgeon but without the explicit knowledge or consent of the patient, performs all or some of the surgery.

Direct and progressive operative experience is considered so essential to the program, that the American Board of Surgery refuses to give complete credit for work done in institutions which do not provide such advancing operative experience and patient responsibility.

How, and to what degree, this problem has vexed the medical profession is best demonstrated by a review of three consecutive actions of the American College of Surgeons' Board of Regents.

On December 7th, 1953, the Board defined ghost surgery as: "That surgery in which the patient is not informed of, or is misled, as to the identity of the operating surgeon."[62]

Dr. Paul R. Hawley, as Director of the American College of Surgeons, in commenting on the definition, reported the following: "The effect of the definition of ghost surgery upon resident training aroused the most concern; yet the Regents decided unanimously that honesty demanded that no exception be made in this respect."[63]

The definition of December 7 provoked sufficient protest to persuade the Regents to modify it five months later, in favor of the residency training programs. The Board presented the following modifications as clarifications of its definition, subsequent to their meeting of May 1, 1954:

> A surgical operation represents a co-operative effort by the responsible surgeon and his assistant. The exact part which each plays during a particular operation may well and frequently does vary. Ghost surgery has been defined by the Regents as 'that surgery in which the patient is not informed of, or is misled, as to the identity of the operating surgeon.'
>
> The Board considers it to be a breach of ethics when any patient who has made an agreement with a surgeon is operated on by another, without knowledge and consent of the patient. However, the Board considers it proper for the responsible surgeon to delegate to his assistant the performance of any part of a given operation, provided the surgeon is an active participant throughout the essential part of the operation. The Board of Regents approves the inclusion of all patients in residency training programs.[64]

This would indeed have appeared to be a clarification rather than a modification had it not, in turn, met with many objections by those who looked upon it as a compromise. As a further development, the Board of Regents, after hearing the advice of a large and representative group of surgical academicians who felt that the original definition of ghost surgery should in no way be modified in favor of residency training, rescinded its modification of May 7, 1954, and on June 4, 1955, simply reaffirmed its earlier definition of ghost surgery as: "That surgery in which the patient is not informed of, or is misled, as to the identity of the operating surgeon."[65]

Subsequently, in 1958, the Judicial Council of the American Medical Association made explicit, detailed, and insistent statements on the question. By paraphrase and repetition the Judicial Council expressed their view as follows:

> Under the normal and customary arrangements with

private patients, and with reference to the usual form of consent to operation, the surgeon is obliged to perform the operation himself, and he may use the services of assisting residents, or other assisting surgeons to the extent that the operation reasonably requires the employment of such assistance. If a resident or other physician is to perform the operation under the guidance of the surgeon, it is necessary to make a full disclosure of this fact to the patient, and this should be evidenced by an appropriate statement contained in the consent.

If the surgeon employed merely assists the resident or other physician in performing the operation, it is the resident or other physician who becomes the operating surgeon. If the patient is not informed as to the identity of the operating surgeon, the situation is "ghost surgery."

An operating surgeon is construed to be a performing surgeon. As such his duties and responsibilities go beyond mere direction, supervision, guidance, or minor participation.

He is not employed merely to supervise the operation. He is employed to perform the operation. He can properly utilize the services of an assistant to assist him in the performance of the operation. But he is not performing the operation where his active participation consists in guidance or standby responsibilities in the case of an emergency.[66]

If unanimity in principle but disagreement in details has beset the surgeons in dealing with this problem, the same has been true of the theologians.

Father Francis J. Connell, C.S.S.R., proposed the case of a residency training program in which the younger man performs a portion of the operation under the watchful eye of an older surgeon. In his comment, Father Connell reviewed the necessity for such delegated procedures in surgical training, and approved of it from a moral viewpoint provided that there was careful supervision on the scene, that the trainee was fully capable to do the task assigned to him without risk to the patient, and that there was no explicit agreement to the contrary between the patient and the surgeon. In regard to the final proviso, Father Connell made the following observations:

In connection with the last condition, it might be asked

if the positive consent of the patient is necessary beforehand to justify the process described. It would seem that this is not necessary. The average person about to undergo an operation presumably trusts the surgeon in charge, leaving it to his discretion to choose what to do by himself and what to assign to be done by others. For everyone knows that in the course of an operation some functions are performed by the assistants. Hence, if the patient lays down no explicit conditions on this matter, I believe that the surgeon in charge may take it on himself to assign some procedures to the younger doctors, always presuming (to repeat) that he strictly supervises the entire operation, and is assured that no harm will come to the patient through the deputation of an assistant to some portion of the surgery.[67]

At about the same time that Father Connell published the opinion just quoted, Father John J. Lynch, S.J., presented the residency training problem in the *Linacre Quarterly*. Father Lynch likewise reviewed the right of the patient to be protected from all unnecessary surgical risk and the right of private patients to require of the contracting surgeon the total personal service which they reasonably expect. It was regarding the latter point, with regard to the presumed consent of the patient for resident participation in the actual surgery, that the views of these two moral professors differed. In contrast to the passage quoted from Father Connell, Father Lynch said:

Consent of the private patient, however, to undergo surgery at the hands of anyone other than the contracting surgeon is a prime requisite for the lawfulness of this practice. Since it does not seem likely that this consent would ordinarily be given by the private patient for a resident actually to operate, presumption of that consent in ordinary circumstances does not seem to be justified.[68]

Moral Comment: In trying to evaluate the current medical and theological thinking on this subject, it should first be pointed out that, on the one hand, the common good demands that hospitals have adequate surgical residency training programs which do in truth demand progressive operative experience and responsibility on the part of the trainee. On the other hand, it is certainly true that every patient, whether paying or indigent, has a right to be protected from all unnecessary surgical risk.

The indigent patient places himself in the care of a government hospital or private hospital with the understanding that these agencies will provide him with adequate facilities and engage for him competent professional care.

The State has an obligation in distributive justice to supply such care for the needy; and the private institution, in certain cases, has such an obligation in charity. Neither of these obligations, however, gives the indigent patient the right to specify that a particular physician render this care, but only the right to expect that the care be adequate and that his physicians be competent. These requirements can be presupposed in an accepted Residency Training Program under suitable supervision.

When a private patient, however, enters into a professional contract with a specified surgeon, the surgery must be performed by the individual surgeon with such assistance as is reasonably required, unless other arrangements are expressed or clearly implied in the physician-patient relationship, which would allow for some additional participation by the resident but only under the direct supervision of the surgeon.

A third type of patient is the individual who voluntarily enters a health insurance plan which provides for specification of medical care by a third party. An example of this would be a College Health Service. In entering such a plan the student becomes analogous to the indigent patient, who has health care provided for him, but the obligation of the physicians is analogous to their contract with a private patient, in so far as the wishes of the College authorities are concerned.

Psychosurgery

Prefrontal lobotomy, as a generic term, is used here to cover the various neurosurgical invasions of the prefrontal area of the brain which have been used in dealing with various types of mental aberration as well as with intractable pain.

Before dealing with the moral implications of these various

procedures, it is necessary to delineate clearly what we mean
by certain terms and concepts connected with the question.

Mental and personality aberrations are classified today under
the general headings of psychoses and neuroses. By neuroses we
understand those relatively minor disorders of the psychic constitution in which personality and the general behavior pattern
remain more or less intact. The psychoses are understood to
embrace those deeper, more far-reaching and prolonged behavior
disorders such as dementia praecox and the manic-depressive
states.

Prefrontal Area: What is sometimes referred to as the prefrontal lobe of the human brain will be recalled as that region
of the frontal lobe which lies anterior to a plane extending from
the coronal suture to the sphenoidal ridge. While various motor
and sensory reactions have long since been localized in the various areas of the cerebral cortex, this prefrontal region has often
been referred to as "the silent area," and its functions have defied
quantitative analysis.

Some hypotheses represent the prefrontal area as the organ of
personality integration. This type of hypothesis would postulate
the area as underlying the complex organization of a person's
distinctive habits of thought, attitudes, traits, and interests: a
kind of mirror in which the self can view itself against the
totality of its own apperceptive background.

Other theories postulate that experience and intelligence, the
bases of behavior, are mediated by this part of the brain, and
that this area is concerned with the projection of the whole
individual into the future, in forecasting the results of certain
activities and visualizing the effects that these actions will have
upon one's self and one's environment. They would hold that
the synthesis of past experience and the assemblage of the various
parts of a problem, with a view to selecting a proper course
from among alternate choices at the completion of each step,
seem to be centered in the prefrontal area.[69]

Thalamus: The importance of the thalamus, which is a large
mass of grey matter located deep in the cerebral hemispheres,
lies in the fact that the gross sensations of pain seem not only

to be mediated through, but somehow also centered in, the thalamus. Moreover this part of the brain is quite definitely, although still somewhat hypothetically, proposed as the center of the emotions. The results of lobotomy clearly indicate this.

Fibers: Beneath the cortex is the mass of fibrous nerve tissues called the white matter. It will be recalled that some of the nerve fibers interconnect the various cortical areas and are called association fibers; while others, connecting the cortical grey matter with the thalamus, are called projection fibers. These latter are seen as the main pathways of interaction between the thalamus and the cortex.

Surgical Techniques: In the early stages of the development of psychosurgery, lobotomy was the only operation. Lobotomy was designed to interrupt the nerve fiber pathways between the frontal lobe and the thalamus.

In the open operation the burr holes were made in the top of the head, and a core of grey and white matter siphoned out, thus revealing the path of the leukotome, especially in regard to the main cerebral blood vessels. Through this pathway the long fibers of the white matter were severed bilaterally, thus breaking the main connections between the prefrontal cortex and the thalamus.

The closed technique consisted in puncturing the orbital plate of the frontal bone with an ice-pick-like instrument, and with a number of carefully measured sweeping motions, severing the fibers. This method was referred to as transorbital lobotomy.

In addition to these operations, interrupting the pathways between the frontal lobe and the thalamus, other procedures were developed, such as topectomy, which consisted in removal of a specified part of the frontal lobe cortex; and the thalamotomy, which destroyed the medial dorsal nucleus of the thalamus.

More recently chemical techniques have been experimentally tried. The basic concept of all of these procedures is fundamentally the same. The various approaches achieve their result by interrupting the pathways between the two stations, or by invading the terminal at either end.

Post-operative Picture: The operation often produced more or less permanent relief from some delusional and most emotional tension states, and an indifference to pain.

Immediately after the operation the patient was usually dazed, indifferent to his surroundings, completely lacking in initiative, and without control over his most ordinary functions. After a period of weeks or months of careful re-education, about one-third of the patients seemed greatly improved, and about one-third manifested an almost vegetative existence.

The path of the leukotome, however, was necessarily less than precise. Too frequently the post-operative effects were drastic and the real hope for personality improvement was quite tenuous. The 1955 Ethical and Religious Directives for Catholic Hospitals incorporated a cautious attitude toward this type of surgery.

"Lobotomy and similar operations are morally justifiable when medically indicated as the proper treatment of serious mental illness or of intractable pain. In each case the welfare of the patient himself, considered as a person, must be the determining factor. These operations are not justifiable when less extreme remedies are reasonably available, or in cases in which the probability of harm to the patient outweighs the hope of benefit for him."

As the scientific community continued to evaluate lobotomy with longer and less assuring follow-up studies, and at the same time new psychotropic drugs were being discovered and electroshock techniques were being refined, the extensive surgical approach to mental illness became so rare in the United States that it is not even mentioned in the 1971 revision of the Catholic hospital directives.

It would seem that this omission of any specific reference to psychosurgery in the 1971 Ethical and Religious Directives for Catholic Health Facilities was a calculated oversight. Although the gross techniques of the mid-century have been all but abandoned in the United States, experimentation with much more refined and sophisticated surgical and chemotherapeutic approaches to psychosurgery are developing and presenting new and as yet undefined moral questions.

The current rapidity of this resurgence is reflected in the frequency pattern of International Conferences on Psychosurgery. The first such conference was held in Lisbon in 1948, the second in Copenhagen in 1970 and the third in Cambridge in 1972.

A great deal of research is being done on the function of minute segments of the limbic system. Surgical trauma has been dramatically reduced by the introduction of electrodes, cold probes, yttrium seeds, radio-frequency heat lesions, etc., in carefully restricted target areas of the brain, thus eliminating the destructive sweep of earlier surgical techniques. In a comprehensive review of these new approaches (now called "leucotomy" rather than "lobotomy"), W. Sweet reports on some dramatic success in cases of phobia, anxiety, obsession, depression and the affective component (when present) of schizophrenia; but twice repeats the caution that it is too soon to know how lasting either adverse or favorable results will be.[70]

While more specific evaluation of even these techniques must await more conclusive medical data, the concept of constantly more refined intracranial modification, whether surgical or pharmacological, opens up even more perplexing moral questions.

Consider the case of a clinically indicated leucotomy in a patient sufficiently disturbed to refuse consent except under the calming influence of psychotropic drugs or electrical stimulation of the brain. Is such consent free or induced, and properly or improperly induced, and in a given case would presumed consent be sufficient anyhow? If the favorable environmental atmosphere of a modern mental hospital, plus the use of ordinary medication, sometimes relaxes the patient enough to leave him amenable to consent, is the light touching of the limbic system with a stronger pharmacological brush substantially more than a change of cerebral environment, or is it very much a different thing? Robert Neville, of the Hastings Center, would seem to think of the brain as a "special environment for the person."[71] And in the case proposed does this "inner environmental change" merely reduce abnormal psychologic pressures and release the power of free choice, or does it impair freedom in the interest of therapeutic manipulation, and how does one really know which?

Induced brain changes raise the frightening sceptre of invasion of the inner personality mechanism itself, and where that road might lead. And yet one might ask if a malfunctioning cranial component is any more "inner" to man than his blood stream or adrenal glands.

The range of established therapeutic approaches to personality disorders is already broad, and careful experimentation is constantly seeking to expand the means to affect and correct the neurological functioning of man's intracranial executive mechanism. Some earlier methods, such as narcosynthesis and general narcotherapy are already phased out. Others, such as electroshock and other convulsive therapies, are being improved by the use of newer drugs and better mechanisms.

Meanwhile as research scientists continue to probe the secrets of the brain and new techniques are gradually transferred from the investigative context into the therapeutic armamentarium, our greatest ethical caution must be that the gentle art of healing never be allowed to become a means of utilitarian personality manipulation. Not unlike the secrets of nuclear fission, the deeper and more refined approaches to psychopathology could be devastating for mankind in unscrupulous hands.

A sound basis for moral evaluation in these matters can still be found in the following words of Pope Pius XII in his address to the First International Conference on the Histopathology of the Nervous System:

> Moreover, in exercising his right to dispose of himself, his faculties and his organs, the individual must observe the hierarchy of the orders of values—or within a single order of values, the hierarchy of particular right—insofar as the rules of morality demand. Thus, for example, a man cannot perform on himself or allow doctors to perform acts of a physical or somatic nature which doubtless relieve heavy

physical or psychic burdens or infirmities, but which bring about at the same time diminution of his freedom, that is, of his human personality in its typical and characteristic function. Such an act degrades a man to the level of a being reacting only to acquired reflexes or to a living automaton. The moral law does not allow such a reversal of values. Here it sets up its limits to the 'medical interests of the patient'."[72]

In addition to this wise basic moral orientation, all of the cautions of proper clinical research merit particular emphasis here.

"Shock" Treatments

The genesis of the so-called "shock" therapies in mental illness seems to have been that schizophrenia and epilepsy were observed to be usually antagonistic to each other, and in the 1930's insulin, metrazol, and electric current were adopted as the principal media of purposefully induced psychotherapeutic convulsions. Electric convulsive therapy has tended to supersede most pharmacological methods of shock therapy because it is easier to administer, easier to control, and eliminates the serious pre-convulsive anxiety associated with metrazol. Sometimes, however, the pharmacological and electric convulsive approaches are combined in treatments.

Complications of treatment still include some danger of temporary damage to the skeletal system by fractures, as well as possible respiratory, cardio-vascular, neurological, abdominal, and nephritic complications. These various complications are usually not of any serious nature, and fatalities are extremely rare under proper management.

Not all types and shades of mental illness respond well to convulsive therapy. Moreover, there are some diseases and physical conditions which are positive contraindications to shock treatments because of the additional danger involved, and in these cases the danger varies with the nature and extent of the organic disease in question.

Moral Aspects: In view of the fact that convulsive therapy is a medically accepted approach to certain types of psychiatric illnesses, which involves an organic invasion with varying degrees of associated danger, the moral questions regarding these procedures are solved, in general, by proper application of the principle of totality.

Regarding the morality of shock therapy in any individual instance, the physician must evaluate the following elements of the case:

1. Is the degree of danger (how serious and how proximate) involved in this individual case in proportion to the need for, or patient-advantages of, this type of treatment?

2. Is there need for, or patient-advantages of, shock therapy instead of less traumatic forms of treatment?

3. Has the requisite permission of the patient or responsible party been obtained?

Hypnotism

Hypnotism, as an attention-precision phenomenon, inducing a state of relaxation ranging from the lethargic to the somnambulistic stage, together with a peculiar susceptibility to suggestion, is becoming more prominent today as a form of analgesic and anesthetic. Aside from its obvious place in the psychiatric setting, it is occupying a place of greater interest in the eyes of surgeons, particularly dental surgeons, obstetricians, dermatologists, and others.

There are certainly instances in which hypnosis, as an anesthetic, has special advantages over the more conventional chemical analgesics and depressants. To mention a few examples: hypnoanesthesia has been used with patients manifesting some peculiar sensitivity to the chemical agents, as well as in the presence of such respiratory, or cardiac disease which would make the usual anesthesia very dangerous. It has been found helpful in severe burn cases where constant and painful dressing changes and debridement are indicated, and the concomitant anesthesia tends to complicate an already debilitated physiologic status. Moreover, certain neurosurgical procedures requiring the conscious cooperation of the patient have been made more feasible by an apt choice of hypnotic procedure.

Moral Aspect: Although induction of the hypnotic state does not seem to include an invasion of tissue, it does involve something of a modification of the consciousness and freedom of the subject.

To the scientific mind, hypnosis is already long since divorced from any connotation of superstition or spiritism. Moreover it certainly should not be used as a form of entertainment or irrelevant and unscientific experimentation.

In addition to the fact that such a modification of the human person is morally contraindicated, except as a means of seeking the good of the whole individual or in legitimate medical experimentation, there are certain dangers attendant upon hypnotism. Although the medical literature represents divergent views regarding the exact nature and extent of these dangers, they certainly merit proper precautionary consideration.

If proper precaution is taken against the recognized, as well as the disputed concomitant dangers, there is no reason, from a moral standpoint, why one cannot recognize indications for the use of hypnosis among the other indications for anesthesia or analgesia.

The most obvious of the dangers referred to above results from the induction of the whole hypnotic state by an insufficiently trained therapist, or its use with border-line psychotics by one not also trained in dynamic psychiatry.

Secondly, one must be aware of the possibility of masking significant symptoms rather than curing the disease.

Disputed dangers revolve around the concept of deleterious effects of too prolonged use of hypnosis, too great personal dependence of the patient on the therapist, inadvisable post-hypnotic suggestion and, in obstetrics, disturbance of the normal mother-child relationship by too deep hypnosis.

Due precaution must be taken against all such risks and possibilities in the use of hypnosis.

Human Experimentation

Human experimentation is an aspect of medicine which has

aroused considerable moral speculation, both on the part of the moral theologians and on the part of the medical profession.

Medicine, of course, is an empirical science, and every difficult case is likely to have some aspects of experimentation in its therapy. In a certain sense, the very idea of a differential diagnosis implies some degree of experimentation. But, it is not in this every day context of medical trial and error that the moral problem arises.

Nor is there any acute moral difficulty in what might be termed the "do or die" experimental procedures, which can be extremely dangerous in themselves and the outcome of which may often be extremely doubtful, when such experimental procedures are employed as a "last ditch stand" in terminal and rapidly deteriorating types of illness.

Such, for example, would be the case of a very delicate and dangerous brain operation on a patient who is already doomed to proximate death due to a brain tumor. In such a case, the patient has really nothing to lose, and everything to gain if the experiment should be successful. Such "one last attempt" procedures, when they hold out some real hope of success, even though it be slim, are obviously acts of wise administration.

The Problem: The real problem arises in the research laboratories, where procedures and remedies which have been tested on experimental animals, must finally be tried on human subjects.

When the experimental procedure is fraught with real danger of serious injury or even death, and the experimental subject is a healthy individual in whom disease must sometimes be first induced; or when the subject, even if already afflicted with some illness, is not in any terminal stage, the morality of such an experiment must be tested against our concepts of man's limited prerogative over human life, and against the basic concepts of right order.

A Definition of Medical Experiment: By the term "medical experimentation" in the present discussion of its moral implications as applied to human subjects is understood those medical or surgical procedures which are recognized to involve some degree of danger, and which are experimentally applied to the individual subject, not so much in his own interest, as in the interest of humanity through the advance of medical science.

The moral implications of this sort of experimentation can vary according to the various methods of procedure on various types of human subjects.

With regard to experiments which are performed upon people who are in good health, we must distinguish between those procedures which merely involve testing the reactions of new and potentially dangerous drugs in the normal human being, and those which also involve the process of first inducing some disease in the healthy individual as part of the experiment.

With regard to experiments which are performed on people who are already ill with reversible disease, we must distinguish between substituting an experimental remedy in place of proven therapies which are available, and proceeding along experimental lines, because there is no proven therapy for the disease.

Finally, with regard to the chronically ill, we must distinguish that type of experimentation which we might call "incidental," in the sense that it is unrelated to the specific illness, or at least not directly concerned with the present malady, but is directed toward some other contribution to medical knowledge.

These are the principal variables of clinical research which are within the context of the experimental procedure. In addition to these, one must likewise evaluate still other moral dimensions if the research subject is an infant, or is mentally defective, or is an inmate of a penal institution.

The need of a careful and even conservative analysis of modern clinical research was highlighted in 1965, when Dr. Henry K. Beecher of Harvard Medical School, a recognized authority on the subject, charged that violations of human values in clinical trials and experimental surgery, too often produce fatal consequences or severe lifetime impairment. Speaking at a science writers' briefing session in Augusta, Michigan, Dr. Beecher cited eighteen examples of experiments on record which he believed were ethically questionable.[73]

Moral Aspects of Human Experimentation

Although human experimentation is as old as the history of man, with reports of the ancient kings of Persia and the Ptolomies in Egypt handing over condemned criminals for scientific experiments, and Galen giving some formalization to scientific medical observation at the beginning of the Christian era, it was not until the seventeenth and eighteenth centuries that modern clinical research began to break through with Lind's work on scurvy and Jenner's clinically controlled studies on the value of vaccination, and the great forward strides of Claude Bernard and Louis Pasteur. And it was only after the Walter Reed experiments with yellow fever had dramatized the broad public health significance of human experimentation, and the Nazi persecutions had shocked the world with the depths of degradation to which clinical research could descend, that codes of ethics for human experimentation began to appear.

In 1946, the Judicial Committee of the American Medical Association presented brief norms to the House of Delegates which were adopted in December of that year and the code of the Nuremburg Military Tribunal followed in 1947. In 1952 Pope Pius XII included norms for experimentation and research in his address to the First International Congress on the Histopathology of the Nervous System, and in 1953 made further observations in his address to the International Office of Documentation for Military Medicine. Norms were likewise proposed by the British Medical Research Council in 1953, by the World Medical Association in 1954, by the Public Health Council of the Netherlands in 1957, and by the World Health Organization in 1962.

From a study of these documents, the following two general principles and three specific rules for human experimentation have been derived.

General Principle I: Medical experimentation which involves a directly intended suppression of an organic function, or the invasion of the organ itself is not immoral for that reason, provided that the organic functional suppression is not of a serious nature—or, at least, if it is extensive is not permanent.

This activity in the service of humanity, considering man in himself and in his relations to other men, would seem to come under the concept of "wise administration," and likewise meet the exigencies of fraternal charity.

Moreover, in his address of September 14, 1952, on "The Moral Limits of Medical Research and Treatment," Pius XII, dealing directly with the principle of totality, spoke as follows:

"The patient, then, has no right to violate his physical or psychic integrity in medical experiments or research when they entail *serious* destruction, mutilation, wounds or perils." (italics added).

General Principle II : Where there is question of a procedure which carries with it considerable danger of serious mutilation, it is evident from the principle of totality that to directly intend such a mutilation or such a procedure, in the interests of medical experimentation is outside of man's restricted and useful prerogative over his own body and is contrary to the imminent teleology of the parts thereof.

Such an act must be looked upon as one of absolute ownership, rather than one of wise administration.

The distinction between administration and ownership here is as difficult to describe as it is important. As the danger connected with the experiment increases, we reach a point where the entire moral object of the act changes, and an act which could have been classified as one of wise administration, and therefore permitted, becomes a completely different act, an act which would be proper only for an absolute owner, and therefore an immoral usurpation of an exclusively divine prerogative.

Administration or Ownership? : Danger can be defined as the objective probability of incurring some evil, and in the realm of medical experimentation we would say that if the objective probability of so compromising the patient's physical or mental well-being and integrity are such that ordinary men would judge the probable risk to be a considerable one, and would consider the probable result as a serious afflction, then this would take the experimental act out of the realm of administration, and put it into the category of ownership.

Rules for Human Experimentation: With these two basic principles in mind, we may lay down certain definite rules for the guidance of medical experimentation on human subjects:

1. The human subject must be made aware of the full extent of the risks involved in the experiment, and he must freely consent to the entire procedure.

This preliminary is explicitly demanded by the American Medical Association in its directives regarding proper procedures relating to human experimentation,[74] and was likewise stressed by Pius XII in the following words:

> In the first place, it must be assumed that, as a private person, the doctor can take no measure or try no course of action without the consent of the patient. The doctor has no other rights or powers over the patient than those which the latter gives him, explicitly, or implicitly and tacitly. On his side, the patient cannot confer rights he does not possess.

2. All safeguards must be employed to protect the patient from injury.

This rule includes the supposition that the experiments have been first tested on animals, that the experimenters are qualified scientists, and that all accessory precautions are at hand to avert danger, counteract harmful effects, or terminate the experiment should the need to do so arise.

The Judicial Committee of the American Medical Association included this second rule under their requirements as follows:

> . . . (2) the danger of each experiment must be previously investigated by animal experimentation, and (3) the experiment must be performed under proper medical protection and management.[75]

3. A dangerous experiment is not to be undertaken unless the results cannot be obtained by other methods of study and no experiment should be undertaken when there is real reason to believe that death or serious injury will result.

The reasoning behind this third rule is based on the fact that the danger connected with a legitimate experiment is not intended by the experimenters. Precisely as danger, it in no way contributes to the good accomplished by the experiment, and thus, in its moral aspect, it can be approached under the principle of double effect. And under this principle one cannot reasonably permit an evil effect if the intended good can be reasonably obtained in some other way.

Moreover, in the application of the principle of double effect in medical experimentation, there must be a special emphasis on the need to evaluate the proper proportion between the good intended and the evil permitted.

Certainly some experiment-connected danger may be permitted, but it must be remembered that the proportion here is between the good accruing to the commonweal in general, through the advance of medical science, and the evil of the danger of injury to an individual member of society.

In estimating the proportion between the good thus intended and the evil permitted, the scale is already heavily weighted in favor of the individual subject of the experiment; and a possible contribution to the common good, though not without its importance, weighs lightly against serious harm to a given individual. This is so because society in general, or the common good, exists for the individual, not *vice versa*. It is true that in the event of impending common catastrophe, the common good prevails over the individual good; but this is only because the common good must be preserved in the interest of many individuals, and not because the common good is an end in itself.

Moreover, once the danger has reached that degree of seriousness which makes the experimental act cease to be one of administration and begin to be one of absolute ownership, there can be no question of applying the principle of double effect at all, since the moral object of the act itself has become evil.

An Invalid Distinction: The various secular codes of morality regarding medical experimentation, such as the directives of the American Medical Association and the decisions of the Nuremburg Medical Trial, agree substantially with the three basic rules listed above. Some of these secular codes, however, while condemning the type of experiment wherein there is reason to believe that death or disabling injury will result, strongly imply that even these might be permitted, provided that the experimenting physicians themselves also serve as subjects. This distinction is completely illogical, as Pius XII has pointed out in the following words:

> What pertains to the doctor with regard to his patient is equally applicable to the doctor with regard to himself. He is subject to the same broad moral and juridical principles as govern other men. He has no right, consequently, to permit scientific or practical experiments which entail serious injury, or which threaten to impair his health to be performed on his person; and to an even lesser extent is he authorized to attempt an operation of experimental nature which, according to authoritative opinion, could conceivably result in mutilation or suicide. This also applies, moreover, to male and female nurses, and to anyone who feels himself disposed to offer his person as a subject for therapeutic research. . .[76]

In 1959 the National Conference on the Legal Environment of Medicine included the following similar comment in its report: "Paragraph 5 of the Nuremburg Code reads: 'No experiment should be conducted where there is an *a priori* reason to believe that death or disabling injury will occur; except, perhaps, in those experiments where the experimental physicians also serve as subjects.' The phrase: 'except, perhaps, in those experiments etc.' is irrelevant in view of the following: If an experiment is morally contraindicated under basic human considerations as wrong, the participation of the investigator would not morally rectify it."[77]

Clinical Research and Mentally Incompetent Populations: The use of retarded children and other mentally incompetent individuals as subjects for medical research poses an additional problem because of their inability to give an informed consent. While their confinement in a controlled environment and their frequently sound physical health make them ideal subjects for research, their status of mental incompetence, frequently as wards of the state, make many research teams very sensitive to the danger of any violation of human rights in such projects.

The difficulty is a very practical one, and the only answer which seems consistent with the proper concept of the dignity and worth of any human life is fairly obvious, but quite restrictive. No procedure should be undertaken without the consent of the next of kin or other responsible agent, and then only those procedures should be admitted which are very minor, entirely safe, and minimally uncomfortable. In general, the procedure should be such that one would expect any competent patient to give immediate and unhesitating consent for them. This restriction should be followed most faithfully, unless the experimental procedure is designed, in its immediate context, to help this particular patient. In this latter case the ordinary norms of human experimentation could be followed and the consent of the patient could be presumed, unless such consent has been explicitly denied by the next of kin.

Clinical Research on the Unborn: The utilitarian and impersonalistic attitude toward the unborn child which pervades large segments of the American culture today and is disasterously confirmed by the Supreme Court's rulings on abortion presents particular problems in regard to fetal experimentation. In view of the fact that the Catholic Church has always taught and defended what became the basic principle of American democracy, that, "all men are created equal and endowed by their Creator with certain unalienable rights" (a principle which American democracy itself has lately compromised), Catholic ethical guidelines in regard to fetal experimentation need be neither more nor less than those outlined above.

High-risk pre-natal experimental procedures are properly undertaken only in those individual cases in which such procedures are a last available measure to try to save the life of the unborn child. Such are more aptly considered to be proportionate therapeutic risks than experimental procedures.

Total interdiction of clinical research on the unborn is obviously unrealistic and too broad. Much of the research in fetology is mainly observational and minimally procedural. The same norms that apply to any research population which is unable to give explicit consent (such as infants or the mentally retarded) apply here: no experimental or research procedure should be undertaken, unless the danger is so remote and the discomfort so minimal that a knowledgeable subject would be presupposed to give ready consent. This norm applies to the research protocol itself. There is also, of course, the necessity of consent of the parent and conformity with the civil law.

Other questions have been raised regarding the use of dead fetuses in research and teaching. There is, intrinsically at least, no moral dimension here beyond the ordinary autopsy proprieties. Some proposed regulations would prohibit teaching or research procedures on aborted fetuses, unless the abortion had been clearly spontaneous. While such a distinction would not be germane to the ethics of a Catholic hospital, it might concern an individual Catholic working in a public institution. Those who advocate the restriction seem to do so as an affirmation of the malice of induced abortion, or as a caution lest the desire for such fetal material prompt even more frequent abortion. Such reasoning seems inadequate. While restriction would limit valuable research, it is doubtful that the lack of it would encourage abortion. Nor is there any implied approval of crime in the use of autopsy materials derived from the bodies of those who have died as a result of murder or some other crime. Here again, of course, one must be aware of legal restrictions as well as the need for permission of the next of kin.

One further question related to research on the human fetus concerns experimental studies involving fecundation *in vitro*. The various modalities of artificial insemination and their evaluation in Catholic teaching are examined in chapter six. Experimental manipulation of pre-natal human life has rapidly advanced from successful attempts at *in vitro* fecundation with brief survival through the blastocyst stage and beyond, to the use of artificial placentas. Goals are being pursued toward *in vitro* human fecundation with subsequent transplantation into a maternal womb, with some reports of dramatic success.

As will be explained more fully in chapter six, the incompatibility of these research efforts with Catholic moral teaching arises from the evident holiness of marital intercourse as a most sacred and intimate act of mutual self-giving and the uniquely befitting human concurrence in the divine act of creation, in bringing forth new human life. Fecundation *in vitro* desolates the deepest human and personalistic values for a strictly utilitarian laboratory procedure, where the scriptural beauty of "two in one flesh" and the deepest fruition of human love are reduced to the precincts of a petri dish. Moreover, this is to say nothing of the already noted clinical restriction on human research prohibiting experimentation which gravely endangers the experimental subject: in this case, the new life that is conceived.

Clinical Research and Prison Populations

The recently growing involvement of the inmates of federal prisons in research projects indicates the timeliness of the ethical questions peculiar to this context.

The purposes of the incarceration of convicted criminals can be listed as fourfold. The first two: punitive and reformative, are directed more immediately to the criminal himself; while the second two: socio-protective and exemplary-deterrent, look respectively to the protection of society and the prevention of crime.

By evaluating medical research on prison volunteers within the context of the parole system, it can readily be shown that it does not necessarily compromise any of these four purposes of incarceration, and that it can indeed advance the reformative process. The presumption of the parole system is that the reduction of time in prison as a reward for good behavior or meritorious service, coupled with the supervision of the parolee after release, are reformative of selected criminals and without undue risk to the social well-being of the community. Participation in clinical research for the benefit of humanity can certainly be classified as meritorious service, and has been shown frequently to be the occasion of reawakening of self respect, personal fulfillment, and a sense of responsible solidarity with society.

There are, however, two important considerations to be made in this regard. The first is that such research procedures must be kept within the same moral limits, with regard to the degree of danger involved, as any other clinical research. In evaluating this, it must be realized that a proper proportion between the individual's human dignity and worth on the one hand, and some possible advance of medical science for the more remote benefit of humanity on the other, would preclude any serious risk of death or disabling injury in the experiment; unless perhaps there was a real hope of averting an immediate grave threat to the common good, which could be averted in no other way. In any case, prisoner-status of the subject does not alter the degree of acceptable risk, since the experimentation cannot justly be part of the punitive aspect of prison life in view of the exposure to not totally predictable risk, and the probability of unequal and ambiguous punitive effects inherent in such a concept.

Secondly, since participation by prisoners in a research project must be a voluntary participation, to which they give a fully informed and free consent, great care must be taken lest the offering of extremely desirable rewards vitiate the true voluntariety of the participants.

Capital Punishment and Clinical Research: Another question, related to, but independent from, the moral propriety of capital punishment itself, concerns the moral propriety of the state decreeing capital punishment by deep anesthesia and permitting concomitant dangerous clinical research on the anesthetized criminal prior to anesthetic death (which might be delayed for hours or weeks) on those condemned criminals who would request that they be allowed to fulfill the capital sentence in this way.

This type of proposal has received rather wide publicity in recent years, particularly under the impetus of J. Kevorkian, M.D., who does not take a stand either for, or against capital punishment but writes: "as long as capital punishment is in effect, there is a far more humane, profitable, and sensible way to implement it.."[78]

The moral issues involved here might be summed up as follows: the state does have the right, under certain conditions, to impose capital punishment and to implement it by those methods which are designed to achieve its punitive and exemplary-deterrent objectives, without exceeding the bounds imposed by proper sense of human decency. One such method: the gas chamber, does approximate the concept of execution by terminal anesthesia.

In this context, it would seem that the state could, at the request of the condemned, officially decree execution by human experimentation under deep anesthesia, culminating in anesthetic death, if not in the experiment itself.

This view, however, is presented as theoretical rather than practical. There is certain human incongruity in the idea of the medical profession participating in this way in the public execution of criminals, even to the extent of being appointed as executioners, notwithstanding the fact that this would be in the interest of clinical research. Moreover the concept of prolonging the terminal anesthesia for days or weeks as the experiment progresses, and the even subconscious overtones of the ideal "human guinea pig" situation realized in the person of a condemned criminal, could scarcely be without the danger of a deleterious, materialistic and dehumanizing influence on the research team, and on the community itself. Thus although what is done and why it is done might be morally defensible, the circumstances necessarily concomitant with the doing of it lead us to regard the act as morally unacceptable in practice.

Vivisection

Vivisection literally means the cutting of a living subject. The ordinary use of the term in medicine and moral theology has come to include any experimentation with drugs or surgical techniques performed upon living animals.

All recognized ethical directions rightly demand that potentially dangerous drugs and surgical procedures in medical experimentation be tested on animals, whenever possible, previous to their use on humans. Moreover such directives provide for the humane treatment of experimental animals. The term "humane" treatment of animals is not meant to convey a groundless fiction which would equivalate animals to human beings and demand that they be treated as such, but rather implies that human beings be rational in their treatment of animals.

Anyone familiar with the history of the vivisection controversies in the United States is aware of the constant battle of scientific researchers to obtain an adequate supply of animals for experimentation, and the untiring efforts of the antivivisectionists to curtail this activity by every possible ruse. Legislators are caught between the powerful antivivisectionist pressure groups and their own responsibility to provide adequate safeguard to the public health by providing for the availability of a proper supply of animals for medical experimentation.

The propriety of animal experimentation for the advance of medical science is based on the natural hierarchy of created things. Man's intellect and free will place him at the peak of visible creation, with other creatures subservient to his needs and legitimate design, and there is no doubt that animal experimentation has greatly benefited mankind. It is only through such experiments that insulin is available for diabetes, liver extract for anemia, cortisone for Addison's Disease and innumerable surgical techniques for many otherwise fatal maladies. Harvey discovered circulation of the blood through animal experimentation, and if the antivivisectionists were to have their way, cancer would remain incurable forever.

The theologian would not agree with those antivivisectionists who speak of the violation of the "rights" of animals, in terms of moral evil, since a creature which lacks reason and personality cannot be said to have rights, in the ordinary meaning of the word.

There is, however, a moral evil discernible in wanton cruelty to animals, in the inflicting of useless and unnecessary pain, since such actions are opposed to the basic obligation which all rational creatures have to act reasonably. Although this evil is not of a grave or serious nature in itself, it can be related to serious moral aberrations in the human personality. St. Thomas also points out that cruelty to animals often leads men to mistreat their fellow men.[79]

Tissue Grafts and Transplants

Tissue grafts and transplants, in the broadest sense of these terms, include any transfer of tissue from one area of the body to another, or from one body to another. Since a number of moral problems arise in connection with the various types of grafts and transplants, we shall consider here these different types, with a moral evaluation of each.

Autografts: The term "autograft" or "autoplastic transplant" means the transfer of tissue from one part of the body to another. Autografts may involve some mutilation of one part of the body in favor of another part, but since these procedures are undertaken only for the good of the whole body, moral questions arising in this type of surgery are immediately solved under the principle of totality. There is no moral objection to this type of surgery even when it is done for purely cosmetic reasons, provided that the risk to the patient is not disproportionate to the desired result and that the motive for undertaking cosmetic surgery is not morally contraindicated (as, for example, to assist a dangerous criminal to escape detection).

Heterografts: The term "heterograft" refers to the transfer of tissue between individuals of different species. We concern ourselves here with the transplantation of tissue from a lower animal to man. Such transplants are called "zooplastic grafts."

Pius XII, on the occasion of his address to a group of eye specialists and delegates of "The Italian Association of Donors of the Cornea" on May 14, 1956, spoke as follows on the question of zooplastic transplants:

> It cannot be said that every transplantation of tissue that is biologically possible between individuals of different species is morally wrong. But it is still less true to say that any heterogenous transplantation which is biologically possible

is not forbidden or is not objectionable. We must distinguish one case from the other and consider what type of tissue or what organ is to be transplanted.

The transplantation of the sexual glands of an animal to man is to be rejected as immoral. On the contrary, the transplantation of a cornea from a non-human being to a human being would not raise any moral difficulty if it were biologically possible and were warranted. If one declared absolutely that transplantation is morally forbidden on the basis of diversity between species, he would logically have to hold that cellular therapy, which is being practiced more and more frequently, is wrong. Living cells are often taken from a non-human being to be transplanted to a human being where they exercise their function.[80]

The directives of this papal pronouncement as applicable to various types of heterografts will be further explored in the following pages.

Static Heterografts: With research scientists and physicians all over the world engaging in studies relating to organic transplantation, heterografts among lower animals have been successfully accomplished in the laboratory to an amazing degree. In the human context, the bone, cartilage, blood vessels and fascia taken from animals and "freeze dried" have been grafted into humans as struts, or mechanical supports, on which the host tissue may build. This static-type graft does not incorporate or grow itself in the human host, but serves only as a supportive structure. There is no moral objection to the static-type of heterograft from animal to man, as described above.

Static Homografts: Transplantation of non-vital anatomic structures and tissues from animal to man, as described above, likewise has its counterpart in the transfer of such tissues taken from the human cadaver to man. Such static homografts or homologous transplants are done most frequently in bone and blood vessel surgery, and in corneal transplantation.

There is nothing morally objectionable in the concept of transplantation of anatomic structures or tissue from a cadaver to a living human being. This is evident from the nature of the graft itself, and is clear from the already mentioned address of

Pius XII to the Eye Specialists. Here the Roman Pontiff enthu-siastically approved this type of homograft, explicitly with re-gard to corneal transplants, and implicitly in the case of other structures.

At the same time Pius pointed out two possible moral dan-gers in this context. First, there is the subtle risk of a psychologi-cally and morally erroneous attitude, which would equivalate the corpse of a human being to that of an animal, or even a mere "thing," an attitude devoid of the respect that is due the body of the dead. Secondly, the removal of anatomic structures for transplantation can become illicit if the rights and sensi-bilities of the nearest of kin, or others charged with the care of the body, are violated.

Vital Heterografts: A vital heterograft is an organic trans-plantation from one species to another, in which the transplant would continue its vital functions, and produce the physiologic effect expected of the specific tissue.

The research problem in this area concerns the ability to alter the response of the host, or to modify the antigenicity of the implant, or to isolate the implant from the host.

Such transplants were unsuccessfully attempted at the be-ginning of the present century, particularly in the area of renal tissue from rabbit, pig, goat, and lamb to man. Interest in these attempts died with the recognition of the immunologic basis of the rejection phenomenon, but has revived with the recent de-velopment of effective immunosuppressive agents.

Clinical urgency and the lack of a suitable human donor prompted the Tulane group to attempt a renal transplant from a chimpanzee to a forty-three year old man in terminal uremia. Two rejection episodes, one at four days and one at four weeks, were successfully reversed. Although this patient died of pneu-monia two months after the surgery, there was ample evidence that the vital heterograft had been essentially successful.[81]

Endocrine therapy, involving the administration to man of naturally produced animal hormones (thyroid extract, adrenal cortical extract, etc.), presents no moral problem. Neither can we envision any moral difficulty in the implantation of the hormone-producing gland itself in the human body, in the event that this became feasible.

Certainly, this type of tissue transplant does not come within the scope of Pope Pius XII's rejection of "the transplantation of the sexual glands of an animal to man."[82] Moreover, even when dealing with glands that are directly generative, such as the ovaries and the testes, the papal condemnation would seem to be aimed at a type of transplantation which would, in some way, envision an act of attempted generation. Estrogens extracted from animal ovaries are now used, without moral objection, in endocrine therapy. It is true that this is merely the isolation of a chemical substance for therapeutic administration, and is not comparable to transplantation of gonads. Nor is it envisioned that the actual transplantation of the gonad would be even a medically desirable substitute for such therapy, as it would be in the case of adrenal and thyroid glands. Even so, if in the future, the ectopic implantation of some gonadal tissue from animal to man were to be shown practicable as a means of restoring endocrine balance, it would not seem to be excluded by previous papal teaching.

Vital Homografts: The most vexing problem in the field of organic transplantation concerns the vital homograft, or homologous transplant *inter vivos,* which is the transplantation of a part of the body of one living human being to another living person.

At mid-century successful kidney transplants between identical twins, together with the research assault on the rejection phenomenon in tissue transplants, accentuated an interest in these vital homografts; and both theology and the civil law were presented with new problems. Theologians questioned how to reconcile the surgical mutilation of the donor with the principle of totality which indicated that, in the framework of right order, the parts of this body were ordered to the good of this body, and in a rather exclusive way. Blood transfusion had presented no real problem because of the immediate natural replacement of this tissue, but the positive excision of a kidney to be transplanted into someone else did present problems.

Some theologians attempted to justify this by an extension of the principle of totality to the moral unity of the human family, but Pius XII made it clear that the principle of totality (which states that the parts of a physical entity, as parts, are ordered to the good of the whole) could not be *reasonably extended* to justify homologous transplantation of organs.

What Pius XII actually said in this regard is of considerable importance today, but for an additional reason. In the context of the current controversy over *Humanae Vitae* and papal statements in general, it is frequently alleged (by those who have evidently not read the document), that Pius XII initially condemned organic transplantation *inter vivos*, but that the practice is now commonly accepted. The occasion of the Pontiff's remarks was an address to a group of Ophthalmologists (May 4, 1956) regarding corneal transplants from cadaver to man. Parenthetically the Pope remarked that he *was not* speaking about transplants *inter vivos* on that occasion, except to point out that an extension of the principle of totality was not the proper approach to the problem. What he said was as follows:

We shall limit ourselves to the religious and moral aspects of the transplantation of the cornea, not between living human beings (of that we shall not speak today), but from the dead body to the living person. However, we shall be obliged to go beyond the strict limits of this topic to speak of certain opinions which we have encountered on this occasion. . . We have also noticed in the printed documentation, another remark which leads to confusion and which we believe we must rectify. To prove that the excision of organs necessary for transplantation from one living person to another is in conformity with nature and lawful, it has been put in the same category as the removal of a particular physical organ done in interest of an entire physical body. In this instance the members of the individual would be considered as parts, and members of the whole organism which constitutes 'humanity,' in the same manner—or almost in the same manner—as they are parts of the individual organism of man. Then it is argued that, if it is permitted, when necessary, to sacrifice a particular member (hand, foot, eye, ear, kidney, sexual gland) to the organism of 'man,' it should likewise be permitted to sacrifice a particular member to the organism 'humanity' (in the person of one of its members who is sick and suffering). The purpose visualized by this manner of argumentation, to heal, or at least to soothe the ailments of others, is understandable and praiseworthy, but the method proposed and the argument on which it is based are erroneous.[83]

Father John R. Connery, S.J., pointed out (*Theological Studies*, vol. 17, no. 4, [Dec. 1956] pp. 559-561) this statement can scarcely be taken as a condemnation of organic transplantation *inter vivos* since the Pope explicitly claimed that he did not wish to speak of that subject, except to rectify a remark which leads to confusion. This confusion was the extension of the principle of totality to organic transplantation. Father John Lynch, S.J., (*Theological Studies*, vol. 18, no. 2, [January, 1957] p. 229) and Father Gerald Kelly, S.J., (*Theological Studies*, vol. 17, no. 3, [September, 1956] pp. 322-344) agreed with this interpretation of the papal statement to the eye specialists.

On the other hand, some minor direct invasions of the human body for the benefit of other individuals had received the approval of papal teaching, as is found in some forms of medical experimentation and blood donations and transfusions. Moreover, the standard moralists had long since approved and identified the obligation of a mother, under certain conditions, to undergo caesarean section for the benefit of her unborn child. This is certainly a directly intended major mutilation for the benefit of another, based on the law of charity. Father Connery, S.J., makes the following interesting observation in this regard:

> Moreover, it is precisely to the principle of charity that moralists appeal in justifying it, and no attempt is made to reconcile it with the principle of totality. Considering this fact, with those mentioned above, I would conclude that while the principle of totality could never be used to justify organic transplantation, neither does it clearly exclude it.[84]

Thus, while not justifying organic transplantation, the principle of totality certainly would seem to put some limits to it. Likewise, although the principle of fraternal charity can be used to justify organic transplantation, neither can this principle be applied without any limitation. Just what the limits are, in either case, is not always perfectly clear. At the present time, however, it seems safe to say that for the sake of charity, the donor of a transplant may directly intend and authorize a mutilation which would not seriously and permanently restrict his functional integrity, or cause a grave risk to his life. Father Gerald Kelly, S.J., summed up the argument in favor of transplantation as follows:

> Organic transplantation is licit, provided it confers a proportionate benefit on the recipient, without exposing the donor to great risk of life, or depriving him completely of an important function. This thesis is proposed as solidly probable, not certain. The principal argument for the opinion is the law of charity, which is based on the natural and supernatural unity of mankind, and according to which one's neighbor is 'another self'.[85]

The current theological view regarding vital homografts is succinctly summarized in Directive 30 of the *Ethical and Religious Directives for Catholic Health Facilities* (November, 1971) as follows: "The transplantation of organs from living donors is morally permissible, when the anticipated benefit to the recipient is proportionate to the harm done to the donor, provided that the loss of such organ(s) does not deprive the donor of life, nor of the functional integrity of his body."

Determination of Clinical Death

A broader problem related to the question of transplants from cadaver to living patient is the question of the determination of the moment of clinical death. In addition to the obvious general importance of this question, it becomes particularly practical in regard to the removal of vital organs for transplant, because of the strict biological time limitations between the death of the donor and the successful transplant.

The clinical advantages of simply removing a vital organ for transplant from an already deeply moribund and terminally unconscious patient with an absolutely negative prognosis are so obvious, and perhaps tempting, yet clearly murderous, that most legislators of anatomical gift acts have stipulated that the transplant team can, in no way, be involved in the terminal care of the patient-donor. Thus the law itself has sought to guard against this immoral utilitarianism, while at the same time declaring its patent criminality.

The very practical legal, moral and clinical problem is that there was a time when definitive cessation of respiration and heart beat were the evident criteria of clinical death. But with the perfection of the heart-lung machine and other mechanical resuscitators, the question arises of the merely mechanical stimulation of the heart-lung system far beyond the point of the actual death of the patient. This makes pertinent such questions as what is death and when can it be said to have occurred?

In the context of Judaico-Christian theology death is often called a "passing," because it is the passing of that spiritual component of the human person into the spiritual mystery of eternal life, subsequent to the definitive disorganization of the human composite: that definitive disorganization which we call death.

Because that mysterious moment defies exact identification, theologians have previously accepted the traditional and obvious medical identification of clinical death as the definitive closing of metabolic life associated with cessation of spontaneous heartbeat. One might speculate on the moment of separation of soul and body (called "theological death") as perhaps not immediate but soon subsequent, and certainly by the time that the body has become the site of extensive corruption.

While this distinction between clinical and theological death has had a theological significance in the administration of the sacraments, it is without clinico-ethical significance in the sense that, for all practical purposes, the passing from the state of moribund life to clinical death, marks the transition from "dying patient" to "cadaver." The brief interim (if there is one) between clinical death and theological death, need place no restraints on either the transplant team or the autopsy procedures. Once clinical death is established, invasion of the cadaver will have no real relationship to the elusive concept of theological death.

Successful artificial stimulation and maintenance of respiration and heart beat have beclouded the question of clinical death. At what point does the object of this artificial stimulation cease to be a human, albeit unconscious and moribund, person and become a cadaver—a heart-lung preparation in a deceased body? The current clinical approach to this question tends to identify clinical death of the brain and nervous system as the death of the patient, even though other functions are still being artificially maintained.

The American Neurological Society, as well as the wider medical community have approached this problem in terms of "brain death" or "the definitive death of the nervous system," in the sense that total and definitive silence in these areas is a conclusive clinical confirmation that death has occurred even while respiration and heartbeat are being artificially maintained. The studies and recommendations of the scientific community toward establishing criteria of death in this context have been highly reasonable and extremely cautious. Perhaps the most significant set of criteria in this matter emerged from the Harvard Medical School in 1968. Prefaced with the caution that these criteria were submitted only as a guide when the diagnosis of death would be questionable, and were not intended to supplant the traditional indications of death in ordinary cases, and stressing that the flat electroencephalogram is viewed as confirmatory, rather than definitive evidence of death (and even this with certain exceptions), the Harvard criteria and other similar documents have received wide acceptance.

Omitting certain minute neurological details, which are important but not necessary for a general understanding of the criteria, the following is submitted as a summary of this approach to the identification of clinical death.

1. That there be total unawareness to externally applied stimuli. Even the most intensely painful stimuli evoking no response whatever.

2. Observations covering a period of at least one hour by physicians are adequate to satisfy the criteria of no spontaneous muscular movements, or spontaneous respiration or response to any stimuli. After the patient is on a mechanical respirator, the total absence of spontaneous breathing may be established by turning off the respirator for three minutes, and observing whether there is any effort on the part of the subject to breathe spontaneously. (The respirator may be turned off for this time, provided that at the start of the trial period the patient's carbon dioxide tension is within the normal range, and provided also that the patient had been breathing room air for at least ten minutes prior to the trial.)

3. Irreversible coma with abolition of central nervous system activity is evidenced in part by the absence of elicitable reflexes. The pupil will be fixed and dilated and will not respond to a direct source of bright light or to pinching the neck. Ocular movement (to head turning and to irrigation of the ears with ice water) and blinking are absent.

As a rule the stretch or tendon reflexes cannot be elicited; i.e., tapping the tendons of the biceps, triceps, and pronator muscles, quadriceps and gastrocnemius muscles with the reflex hammer elicits no contraction of the respective muscles. Planta or noxious stimulation gives no response.

4. Of great *confirmatory* value is the flat or isoelectric EEG. A flat electroencephalogram is not an essential determination but may be used if desired by the individual physician. We must assume that the electrodes have been properly applied, that the apparatus is functioning normally, and that the personnel in charge is competent. It is advised that one channel of the apparatus be used for an electrocardiogram. This channel will monitor the ECG so that, if it appears in the electroencephalographic leads because of high resistance, it can be readily identified. It also establishes the presence of the active heart in the absence of the EEG. Another channel should be used for a noncephalic lead. This will pick up space-borne or vibration-borne artifacts and identify them.

All of the above tests should be repeated at least twenty-four hours later with no change.

The validity of this data should depend on the absence of two elements, which can produce a flat electroencephalogram in the living: hypothermia and certain central nervous system depressants such as barbiturates.

Several State legislatures have recognized the validity of brain and central nervous system death as the death of the individual (e.g., Kansas, Maryland, Virginia) and my own judgment, confirmed in consultation with many theologians, is that these are morally safe criteria, and may be followed in practice for identifying the status of clinical death, both for the removal of vital organs for transplant (the previous permission of the patient being sufficient under the Anatomical Gift Act), and for the discontinuance of mechanical respiration and cardiac stimulation. It is to be carefully noted here that in these adjuncts, we are not dealing with the question of prolongation of life in terminal illness, but with the question of recognizing that death has already occurred.

Surgery/Suppressive Therapy within Generative System

As has already been pointed out, once the object of surgery or suppressive therapy falls within the human generative system, a new moral problem arises.

In such a situation the procedure must not only conform with the principle of totality, but must also be judged in the light of the principle of double effect.

Actually, within the context of the human generative system, there are two distinct effects in the moral order. There is the physical removal of an organ, or the suppression of its function in the interests of the whole body, which must be judged to be in accord with the imminent teleology of the part. This is known as the therapeutic effect, which is viewed in the light of the principle of totality.

In addition to this, however, the removal of a generative organ, or the suppression of its function results in a limitation of the procreative faculty. This is known as the contraceptive effect of the procedure.

If the procedure were undertaken precisely as a contraceptive measure, even though in the interests of the whole body, this would be contrary to Catholic teaching on contraception. This is so because the generative organ, precisely as generative is not, to this extent, viewed as subordinated to the good of the individual.

In the controversial atmosphere following the issuance of the encyclical *Humanae Vitae*, a considerable amount of confusion and error came about, because some writers misinterpreted directives six and twenty of the *Ethical and Religious Directives for Catholic Facilities* in an erroneous attempt to justify directly contraceptive sterilization for clinical indications. Confusion on this point has become so widespread that the question merits some detailed comment here.

Directive Six is found under the "General Directives" and is a brief reminder of the principle of totality. It reads as follows: "Ordinarily the proportionate good that justifies a medical or surgical procedure should be the total good of the patient himself." *Directive Twenty* deals with the distinct moral entity of "indirect sterilization." It follows Directives Eighteen and Nineteen in which the teaching of the Church on "direct sterilization" (as expressed in the encyclical *Humanae Vitae*) is set forth. These directives read as follows: *Directive Eighteen:* "Sterilization, whether permanent or temporary, for men or women, may not be used as a means of contraception." *Directive Nineteen:* "Similarly excluded is every action which, either in anticipation of the conjugal act, or in its accomplishment, or in the development of its natural consequences, proposes, whether as an end or as a means, to render procreation impossible." *Directive Twenty:* "Procedures that induce sterility, whether permanent or temporary, are permitted when: (a) they are immediately directed to the cure, diminution, or prevention of a serious pathological condition and are not directly contraceptive (that is, contraception is not the purpose); and (b) a simpler treatment is not reasonably available. Hence, for example, oophorectomy or irradiation of the ovaries may be allowed in treating carcinoma of the breast and metastasis therefrom, and orchiectomy is permitted in the treatment of carcinoma of the prostate."

The critical concepts which must be clearly understood in the reading of these directives are first, the idea of "direct sterilization" (also sometimes called "contraceptive sterilization") which is forbidden in Directives Eighteen and Nineteen; and secondly, the idea of "indirect sterilization," which is dealt with in Directive Twenty and which is acceptable in Catholic Health Facilities when clinically indicated.

Direct sterilization means that the *purpose* of the procedure is to render the patient *infertile*. This is sometimes desired, either because the patient does not want to have any further pregnancies, or because the physician judges that further pregnancies would be likely to have deteriorating, or complicating effects on some pathological condition such as renal or cardiac disease. The ordinary surgical procedure is to preclude pregnancy by surgically dividing the fallopian tubes, and thus blocking the path of union between ovum and sperm. However clinically feasible this may be, it is a directly contraceptive sterilization, because it directly seeks to bring about infertility, even though only as a means or a step in the therapeutic regimen. It is thus contrary to Directive Nineteen, which is a direct quotation from *Humanae Vitae.*

Indirect sterilization, on the other hand, is described in Directive Twenty. The clinical rationale of indirect sterilization is not precisely to suppress fertility (it would be performed, when clinically indicated, on an unmarried patient: e.g., a priest or a nun, for the same reasons as on a married patient). The rationale is to suppress the endocrine function of the generative organ, because the endocrine function is detrimental to some other pathology (as in ovarian suppression in the presence of cancer of the breast) or to block the path of a retrograde infection (e.g., ligation of the vasa deferentia in some cases of prostate surgery). It is evident that the purpose of the procedure in these cases is not to prevent conception.

Thus, the principle of totality cannot be used to justify direct sterilization, and that is precisely the reason for the word "ordinarily" in Directive Six. Tubal ligation to prevent pregnancy which might complicate some other pathology (such as a renal or cardiac disease) is "direct sterilization" and as such is in opposition to Directives Eighteen and Nineteen. Directive Twenty deals only with "indirect sterilization" and is unrelated to the case presented.

Hence, a sterilization is called "directly contraceptive," when the purpose for which it is done is to prevent pregnancy. The fact that a more ultimate purpose may be considered therapeutic, e.g., to preclude the strain of pregnancy in the presence of cardiac or renal disease, does not make the procedure other than a directly contraceptive one. In such a case it is evident that the procedure must first be contraceptive before it can be therapeutic: i.e., the therapeutic goal is precisely the suppression of fertility.

Again, in March 1975, the Holy See clearly reiterated this teaching in a reply of the Congregation for the Doctrine of the Faith to questions submitted by the Bishops of the United States ("Responses to Questions of the Episcopal Conference of North America: Prot. 2027/69, March 13, 1975). We call attention here to two extremely significant quotations from this reply:

"1. Any sterilization which of itself, that is, of its own nature and condition, has the sole immediate effect of rendering the generative faculty incapable of procreation, is to be considered direct sterilization, as the term is understood in the declarations of the Pontifical Magisterium, especially of Pius XII. Therefore, notwithstanding any subjectively right intention of those whose actions are prompted by the care or prevention of physical or mental illness which is foreseen or feared as a result of pregnancy, such sterilization remains absolutely forbidden according to the doctrine of the Church. . . .

"2. The Congregation, while it confirms this traditional doctrine of the Church, is not unaware of the dissent against this teaching from many theologians. The Congregation, however, denies that doctrinal significance can be attributed to this fact as such, so as to constitute a "theological source" which the faithful might invoke and thereby abandon the authentic Magisterium, and follow the opinions of private theologians which dissent from it."

The usual surgical approach to contraceptive infertility is by ligation of the fallopian tubes of the female, or the vasa deferentia of the male, or by irradiation of the gonads, or even hysterectomy or oophorectomy. Temporary pharmacological contraceptive infertility is achieved by hormonal suppression of ovulation or spermatogenesis, or by modification of the female cervical mucus.

The moral aspects of contraception in general, and of contraceptive sterilization in particular, are treated in chapter six. The matter under consideration here, on the other hand, includes various pharmacological and surgical procedures which result in sterility, but which are not done with contraceptive intent, and hence are not properly called directly contraceptive procedures. The infertility which is foreseen as their side effect is neither the purpose for which they are done, nor their sole immediate effect. Hence these procedures are properly evaluated under the principle of double effect.

Primary Gonadal Pathology: Perhaps the most evident examples of indirect sterilization are found in those cases in which serious pathological lesions of the gonads themselves indicate surgical castration by oophorectomy or orchiectomy, such as cancer of the ovary or testis. Such cases are classical examples of the proper application of the principle of double effect, insofar as the resulting sterility is clearly a side effect of the therapeutic procedure, the radical approach is likely to be considered clinically imperative, and the proportion between the loss of the generative function and the extirpation of the dangerously pathological tissue is evident. A similar example could be found in a dangerous menorrhagic condition in which an approach less radical than definitive surgery, such as temporary pharmacological suppression by hormonal therapy, would not be considered feasible.

Ovarian Radiation and Breast Cancer

Irradiation or surgical extirpation of healthy ovaries is permitted in certain types of fulminating breast cancer, if the resulting inhibition of hormonal activity is expected to retard the spread, or post-operative recurrence of the cancer; or irradiation of, or removal of, the testes in carcinoma of the prostate is sometimes done in order to inhibit cancer growth by abolishing the testicular hormonal activity.

With regard to these latter cases, the following words of Copeland are very much to the point:

> Malignant tumors which most frequently metastasize to bone arise from the prostate and the breast. The organs are intimately related functionally to the male and female gonads. The relationship of cancer to hormonal stimulation or control is now receiving intensive study, and, in the breast and prostate gland, it is well known that a hormonal imbalance will affect cancer growth in these organs or in their metastases. The exact mode of action by the hormones has not been definitely established, but the real effect on the rate of growth of the malignant cell is indisputable. Changes in the hormonal environment of tumor cells from organs intimately related functionally to the gonads, seem to affect the growth potential of these tumor cells. Such a change in environment can be brought about by castration and/or adrenalectomy, suppression of gonadal activity by the administration of the appropriate antagonistic sex hormone; or by increasing the amount of the existing sex hormones with supplemental dosage.[86]

Regarding this type of castration for cancer of the breast, it would not seem admissible (even under the principle of double effect) in the presence of pregnancy, with subsequent loss of the fetus. Although such a procedure would technically be an "indirect abortion," its justification would be most doubtful because the need and efficacy of the ovarian suppression seems to be somewhat uncertain, and hence not proportionate to the loss of the fetus. Hugh Miller, for example, reviewing sixty-five instances of cancer of the breast during pregnancy, concluded that: "There is no proof that surgical or radiation suppression of ovarian function influences survival rate."[87]

Vasectomy and Prostatectomy: The surgical procedure of double vasectomy immediately prior to prostatectomy as a prophylaxis against epididymitis is an operation which has been practical for the past seventy years.

The enucleation of the prostate leaves the way open for post-operative infection to spread rapidly within the lumen of the seminal vesicles and the vasa deferentia. Although other mechanics of sepsis are described, the above is generally accepted as the most common route of the retrograde infection.

Dividing the vasa deferentia interrupts the path of infection. The incidence of epididymitis after prostatectomy reaches up to 20% without vasectomy, whereas with vasectomy the complication is almost eliminated.[88]

Epididymitis is a painful complication and, in the older age group, not without some dangers such as increased susceptibility to infection, lowered general resistance, and increased risk of atelectasis, thrombophlebitis, and pneumonia, due to the protracted nonambulatory state of the patient.

In the moral evaluation of the procedure we must first recognize that, from the very nature of the case (a prophylactic procedure to prevent the spread of infection), the resultant sterilization is not directly intended, but merely foreseen and permitted. Hence, as a therapeutic rather than a directly contraceptive procedure, the operation does essentially come under the principle of double effect.

The liceity of a procedure is not immediately established by the fact that the evil effect (sterilization) is merely permitted and not directly intended. We must also look to the proportion betweeen the good effect and the evil effect, and question whether the good effect can be reasonably obtained in some other way without the concomitant evil effect.

It is this required due proportion that demands a selection

of cases for vasectomy in prostatectomy. In the older age group of patients, whose fertility may be waning, and in whom the complications of epididymitis are more serious, the vasectomy can be performed without moral objection. The procedure is, however, clearly contraindicated, from a moral viewpoint, in the younger age group or in any male who is still well within the period of his fertility.

The Falk Procedure: The Falk procedure is described as a cornual resection of the fallopian tubes in the presence of recurrent salpingitis due to recurrently exacerbating gonorrheal infection. The infection is implanted from below, invading by way of the cervix and reaching the tubes by direct extension along the endometrium of the uterus, and it is believed to be self-limited in the tubal area. The purpose of the Falk procedure, therefore, is to break the uterine-tubal pathway, thus permitting the healing of the tubal inflammation and at the same time blocking the avenue of any recurrent gonorrheal infection insofar as the tubes are concerned. This procedure, moreover, by leaving the tube in situ, is designed to conserve the ovarian blood supply.

Disagreement among physicians regarding the advisability of the Falk procedure has not helped the theologians arrive at a clear cut analysis of the morality of the operation.[89]

Although the procedure is seldom used today, the Falk technique is an intriguing one, since it represents a case of tubal ligation which is not a directly contraceptive sterilization. The operation as described above evidently does not envisage the suppression of the generative faculty, precisely as generative, either as a means or as an end, since its sole purpose is to divide the pathway of a migratory infection, and its prophylactic value is in no way enhanced by its contraceptive result.

But again the fact that a therapeutic procedure is accompanied by a foreseen but unintended contraceptive effect, and can be thus essentially fitted into the framework of the principle of double effect, does not immediately tell us that the procedure is permitted.

For the consideration of the proportion between the good

effect and the evil effect in this case, one must remember that gonorrheal infection of the cervix accounts for about 60% of all acute pelvic inflammatory disease.[90]

Moreover, it seems that reinfection by no means depends on renewed sexual contact, but the gonorrheal focus can be a constantly smouldering infection in the cervix, with periodic flare-up into endometritis. As the infection again travels along the uterine endometrium and into the tubal area, one is not confronted with just an infected set of fallopian tubes, but the angry tube becomes occluded and distended, and the purulent exudate may escape from the distal end, giving rise to acute pelvic peritonitis and pelvic abscess, as well as adhesions at the site of the adjoining pelvic structures, or between these and the small intestine, sigmoid, and rectum.

In such a situation the tube is so occluded that the patient nearly always is, or soon will be, sterile; and still subject to further pelvic devastation by the recurrent infection.

Since the therapeutic and prophylactic effect of the Falk procedure is to isolate the infected tubal area, allowing the self-limited infection to subside and breaking the pathway to re-infection, and since whatever contraceptive result there may be (if the lumen of the tube still has any patency), will only be anticipating a soon to be expected sterility due to infection-occlusion, there is evidently an acceptable proportion between the good effect and the evil effect, from the moral viewpoint.

As regards the other requirement of the principle of double effect: that the good effect cannot be reasonably achieved in some other way, without the concomitant evil effect, it must be pointed out that antibiotic therapy has not been dramatically effective against the sophisticated gonococcus. Antibiotic therapy, in the circumstances described above, would be, to say the least, a much less effective and secure way of combating the particular situation: while adding little or no hope for sufficient patency of the tubal lumen to achieve fertility.

In view of these considerations, we would say that the Falk procedure is definitely not a directly contraceptive sterilization, and that if it is gynecologically indicated the surgeon may safely proceed, from a moral viewpoint, under the principle of double effect.

Myomas and Hysterectomy: A myoma is described as any tumor which is made up of smooth muscular elements. The presence of myomas beneath the uterine mucosa (submucous myoma) is mentioned here because some physicians have considered this condition a real contraindication for pregnancy, and perhaps too frequently, a sufficient indication for hysterectomy, particularly in the presence of bleeding. The following observations of Welch are significant:

> Hysterectomy of any sort—total, subtotal or vaginal—is a tried and true treatment for myomas of the uterus. While it is the commonest operation used in this condition, it falls short of the desired goal in young women in whom preservation of the reproductive function is so important. Hysterectomy, in general, is justified when the prevailing circumstances or pathologic aspects outweigh a reasonable chance or desire of reproduction.[91]

The question of hysterectomy for myomas was submitted to the "Queries and Minor Notes" department of the Journal of the American Medical Association as long ago as May 1957. Two consultants who responded to the question in the Journal supply us with a medical answer which is still morally sound:

> The possibility of myomectomy immediately suggests itself if the bleeding is debilitating or if the tumors are growing rapidly. It is possible to remove many fibromyomas, including submucous, and preserve a uterus that is capable of impregnation and maintaining pregnancy . . . the most radical procedure would be complete hysterectomy, but it is hoped that this would not be necessary . . . There does not seem to be any reason that pregnancy should not be attempted.[92]

Sometimes the medical literature reflects the opinion that, although extensive uterine myomas can constitute an indication for hysterectomy, conservatism and the greater good of the patient is perhaps occasionally sacrificed in pursuit of a line of least resistance. To cure without deformity or loss of function is not only the surgeon's ideal, but often his basic obligation.

Discussing myomectomy and hysterectomy before the New York Obstetrical Society in 1958, Lordaro said of myomectomy: "In general it is a more difficult and painstaking procedure than hysterectomy. It requires more thought, greater fortitude and technical skill, and, above all, patience . . ." And while allowing for the fact that some cases definitely require hysterectomy, the same specialist significantly added: "Physicians have no right to decide arbitrarily when a woman should cease to bear children."[93]

It should be noted here that myomectomy *during* pregnancy can sometimes become a necessity in the presence of acute degeneration of fibroid tumors. The procedure is not without considerable danger, to the fetus more than to the mother. It should be undertaken only when absolutely necessary, and according to the element of proportion of attendant danger and hope of safety for both mother and child, according to the principle of double effect.

Endometriosis: Endometriosis is described as a condition in which tissue more or less perfectly resembling the endometrium, or lining of the uterus, is found abnormally distributed in the uterus itself or ectopically in the ovaries, Fallopian tubes, uterine ligaments, adjacent peritoneum, cervix, vagina and/or recto-vaginal septum. Sometimes such endometrial tissue is found in other pelvic areas, such as the bowel, the bladder and the ureters, the perineum, the umbilicus, and the vulva. Even the upper arm, the back of the thigh, and the pleura have been authentically described as sites of endometriosis.[94] The classical pelvic endometriosis is frequently accompanied by retroversion of the uterus with uterine adherence to the rectum. Since the aberrant endometrial tissue usually responds to the hormone-induced changes of the menstrual cycle, pain at the ectopic sites is accentuated at menstruation. Pregnancy causes the problem to regress, and the subsequent improvement is sometimes sustained after the pregnancy for periods up to three or four years.

Beecham made the following interesting observations in this regard:

Nature has employed an efficient prophylactic and curative measure for endometriosis, i.e., pregnancy. It is note-worthy that the frequency with which the diagnosis of endometriosis is made, parallels the increased use of contraception, the emancipation or rise of womankind to careers and/or late marriage with late childbearing.[95]

Moral Comment: Some moral comment on the treatment of endometriosis is in order, since the physician is faced with the choice of inducing sterility by a surgical or radiological approach, thus eliminating the monthly exacerbation of the disease, or by tedious dissection of the ectopic endometrial tissue, with hope of substantial success, but with the possibility of the need for further surgery after some years; or by the newer pharmacological approach of hormone-induced temporary pseudo pregnancy.

Emphasis on both types of surgical treatment, radical and conservative, can be found in the medical literature. The radical approach, with its subsequent sterility, would certainly be indicated in some extreme cases, and would be completely defensible under the principle of double effect.

But those cases wherein there is real hope of preserving or reactivating the childbearing function by conservative surgery require further careful moral consideration. Even though the therapeutic result of conservative surgery might be somewhat limited and further surgery might be later indicated, one could not defend radical surgery under the principle of double effect without a real necessity of sacrificing the childbearing function as the only avenue to reasonable remission of the disease. This is because it would be difficult to identify the proper proportion between the two effects, in view of the fact that the hypothetical need for subsequent surgery would not be realized in many cases.[96]

Aside from the surgical approach, attempts have been made to induce a pseudo-pregnancy by administration of hormones, thus bringing about anatomical changes similar to pregnancy. The rationale of the treatment is that the beneficial effects of pregnancy on endometriosis are thought to result from the inhibition of ovulation.[97]

Among a number of reports on this regimen, that of Lebherz and Fobes (Bethesda Naval Hospital) is both typical and
significant. Reviewing 112 cases of endometriosis treated with
the newer progestational steroids (norethynodrel and more-
thindrone) they reported:

> We feel that norprogesterone does affect ectopic endo-
> metrium favorably from the host's standpoint and can be
> expected to produce subjective and objective relief both
> during and after therapy in 75 to 80 per cent of cases. Since
> long-term follow-up is not yet available, duration of therapy
> is prolonged (nine months), and troublesome side effects do
> occur, use of this drug for conservative management of
> endometriosis should at present be restricted to symptomatic
> patients, thirty-five years and younger, especially where
> childbearing is to be considered.[98]

The clinical details of this type of regimen will undoubtedly
clarify as it continues to be used.

From a moral viewpoint, this long term induction of the
sterile state would not be a directly contraceptive measure, but
rather a therapeutic suppression of the menstrual endocrine pattern. This presents itself as a functional suppression of the
generative system precisely as part of the body, and not in its
generative role, and would be morally unobjectionable.

Hysterectomy for Prolapse of the Uterus: Prolapse, which
merely means a downward displacement or sinking, can affect
the uterus of the female patient at almost any age. The usual
classification admits of three degrees of uterine prolapse, varying
from a slight descent to the extreme condition referred to as
"procidentia," in which the entire uterus protrudes through
the vagina. The discomforts and dangers of fatigue, ulceration
of the cervix and vaginal mucosa, plus bowel and urinary difficulties accompany prolapse to a greater or less degree.

The problem, with regard to uterine prolapse, which engages
the attention of the moralist can be indicated without going
into further technical descriptions of the anatomical pathologies
involved. While prolapse of the uterus is widely listed as one of
the standard indications for hysterectomy, there is a noticeable

trend in the literature toward conservative repair of the difficulty in patients still in their childbearing period.

The most popular repair is the Manchester-Fothergill operation (or some variation of this technique) which includes the
plication of the fascia of the anterior vaginal wall, amputation
of the cervix, shortening of the cardinal ligaments, and a high
posterior vaginal wall repair. After the repair, pregnancy may
successfully be carried to term, although caesarean delivery is
usually indicated.

Moral Comment: In those cases where there is hope of effective repair and reasonably good conservation of the childbearing
function, and the patient indicates her desire for further fertility,
or her reluctance to sacrifice her menstrual function, it would
be morally wrong to resort to hysterectomy for uterine prolapse. If the patient, however, wishes hysterectomy, not as a
convenient contraceptive, but rather for her own future well
being and the avoidance of further pelvic problems, her desires
should be respected. Such an attitude, in most circumstances
of prolapse, would not be morally reprehensible. In other words,
the patient, in her role as administrator of her own body, while
having a definite obligation to protect and conserve her childbearing function, is not always obliged to take every possible
means to do so. If she is normally obliged to use only ordinary
means to prolong life itself, then there is certainly some room
for discretion in what means she must use to preserve an individual function. The trauma and expense of conservative surgery,
with the likelihood of a less than fully satisfactory result and a
future need for more extensive surgery, may not be proportionate to the temporary preservation of her fertility.

Obviously, in an individual case, it is not for the theologian
to decide whether more extensive or conservative surgery should
be done. This is an obstetrical question depending for its answer
on the details of each case, on the prudent judgment of the
gynecologist and, not least, upon the reasonable wishes of the
informed patient. Theology can only indicate the moral considerations which should enter into the decision.

Unjustified Hysterectomy: In dealing with the question of

surgery within the generative system, a medical moral treatise must contain some reference to the problem of unjustified hysterectomy. The testimony of the medical profession itself leaves no doubt as to the magnitude of abuse in this area, but that very testimony is likewise a heartening sign that the same profession is alert to the abuses, and striving to correct them.

No one can find fault with the relatively small percentage of unnecessary hysterectomies which are recognized as unnecessary only in hindsight, and which were done with reasonable indication that more extensive surgery was the safest procedure.

But it is the hysterectomy which is done, as Wharton points out, because: "This is often the path of least resistance both for the physician and patient,"[99] which casts some shadow on the high ideals of the medical profession. And most unfortunately, the known truth behind even conservative statements like the following is a disgrace which some few have inflicted upon the good name of the medical profession.

"There has been a gradual increase in the number of vaginal hysterectomies performed during the last few years. This has been chiefly due to a desire to familiarize residents with the technique of this procedure, and to a lesser extent to the broadening of indications for vaginal hysterectomy."[100]

Elective Hysterectomy Following Bilateral Oophorectomy : When some pathologic condition of the ovaries necessitates their surgical excision, the gynecologist may frequently wish to remove the uterus and its other adnexa at the same time, although these other organs are perfectly normal. The reason for this type of elective hysterectomy is the desirability of leaving a "clean pelvis" as a prophylactic measure against possible future pelvic complications. Note the following quotation from Te Linde:

> When all the adnexa are removed it is our custom to perform a hysterectomy, unless there is a very good reason for conserving the uterus. The pelvis is usually more easily peritonealized after removing the uterus, which often is covered with shaggy adhesions. Furthermore, a possible source of leukorrhea and malignancy is thereby removed.[101]

Moral Comment: Elective hysterectomy, as it is described here, presents no real moral problem. In most situations (such as pelvic inflammatory disease or malignant lesions of the ovaries) there will be clear positive medical indication for removing the already affected uterus. But even in those cases where there is no present uterine involvement, the surgeon's desire to leave a "clean pelvis" certainly offers a reasonable cause to undertake the incidental removal of a now-functionless uterus provided he has the expressed or implied consent of the patient. Since the reproductive function has already been necessarily sacrificed, the principle of double effect would not be invoked, but only the principle of totality. The hysterectomy is understood to involve no real additional surgical risk, and since it would in no way additionally impair the functional integrity of the patient, the desirability of a "clean pelvis" would certainly justify the procedure.

Elective Oophorectomy: In view of the hormone-secreting aspects of the ovaries as endocrine glands, the question of elective oophorectomy (when hysterectomy is indicated) is not quite as simple as that of elective hysterectomy. The question is usually raised only in regard to the patient who is near the menopause, or is post-menopausal. Most gynecologists would not consider removing non-pathologic ovaries in a woman much below the age of forty, since the endocrine balance is desirably maintained, unless there is one positive indication for oophorectomy or irradiation, such as cancer of the breast.

But even regarding the patient near or after the menopause, there is no unanimity among physicians regarding elective oophorectomy. Two of the most distinguished American gynecologists, Te Linde and Wharton of Johns Hopkins, comment as follows:

> The uterus for many years, in numbers now probably astronomical, has been removed in toto or in part. On some occasions the ovaries are also removed, at other times they are allowed to remain. One would think that by 1960 the effect of the removal of the uterus on the ovary and its function would be clear and not a subject of controversy; yet, this is not the case.[102]

These authors go on to say that although some distinguished physicians are of the opinion that the interest of the patient is best served by bilateral oophorectomy, they themselves lean toward the advisability of conserving ovarian tissue after hysterectomy.

Edmund Novak and Tiffany Williams made a significant contribution to this question by reviewing the pros and cons of the elective procedure, from those who hold that hysterectomy at any age should be followed by castration because of the likelihood that degenerative changes in the ovarian tissue will soon render these organs functionless, through those who advocate the total operation after the age of forty as a prophylactic measure against the possibility of future ovarian cancer, to those who minimize the danger of ovarian cancer and stress the role of the ovary in endocrine balance and psychologic stability even after the climacteric.[103] And although the current medical literature seems to reflect a growing tendency toward the conservation of ovarian tissue in these circumstances, in such controversial gynecological questions the theologian can only try to help the physician interpret the evidence in the light of the principle of totality, and the total fulfillment of the patient as a human person. Indeed, for example, at times the physician may judge that a particular patient is so unlikely to have regular pelvic examinations in the years subsequent to hysterectomy that this, in itself, might be a valid indication for the additional procedure of prophylactic oophorectomy.

Uterine Damage in Multiple Caesarean Sections

A particularly difficult moral problem with regard to hysterectomy can arise after multiple caesarean sections, as is demonstrated in the following case:

A woman who has already undergone several caesarean sections is again pregnant. The doctor judges that this time he will be unable to repair the uterus in such a way that it will safely support another pregnancy. He wonders, therefore, if, during the course of the coming caesarean section, he finds this judgment to be verified, he may remove the uterus.

The precise difficulty in this case arises from the fact that some of the theologians who have dealt with it have considered the radical procedure described above as an act of directly contraceptive sterilization, on the grounds that such a uterus at rest does not constitute any danger to life; and that the danger arises only if the woman should again become pregnant; and that since the uterus is being removed with a view to preventing this contingency, the operation is one of directly contraceptive sterilization.

Classical Moral Opinion: The classical moral theologians do not appear to handle the problem exactly as it is presented in the above case. Their treatment covers only the two extreme cases; namely: the mutilation of a healthy generative organ to prevent a pregnancy, which would be dangerous because of a concomitant disease in some other organ outside the generative system, such as the heart or lungs; or, at the other extreme, the destruction of a generative organ which is itself affected by some disease, such as cancer, and is subject to an invading pathology which is quite independent of its generative function, and which must be radically remedied at once.

Of these two extreme cases, the first is evidently a directly contraceptive sterilization, and the second is equally evidently a directly therapeutic sterilization. The problem which concerns us here is different from both of them: the damaged uterus is not a healthy organ, but neither does it involve danger to life independently of its function.

Contrary to the opinion of those referred to above, who maintain that radical surgery in this case is a directly contraceptive sterilization, we maintain, at least as a solidly probable opinion, that the uterus may be removed in these circumstances, and that such removal is a directly therapeutic procedure.

The More Strict Opinion: No one would deny the fact that a dangerously pathologic organ, in view of the principle of totality, may be removed. Those who hold the stricter opinion simply maintain that the uterus, in its present condition, is not dangerously pathological, that the cause of the danger is the fact of a future pregnancy, that this danger can be averted by abstinence or periodic continence, and that to remove the uterus here and now is a directly contraceptive procedure, because it is aimed at averting a future danger which would only arise from a future pregnancy.

The Less Strict Opinion: The more liberal view, on the other hand, maintains that since an organ is essentially functional rather than static, there is a certain ineptitude in speaking of an organ as dangerously pathologic, or non-pathologic, except in terms of its function.

Granting that the patient is not in imminent danger until the uterus undertakes its primary function of pregnancy, those who defend the more liberal opinion would maintain that the cause of the danger lies within the damaged uterus itself, and that the fact of pregnancy is rather the occasion, or at most a partial cause, of the danger to life.

Hence, they would hold that here and now the uterus, even in the nonpregnant state, is properly referred to as a functionally dangerously pathological organ.

In view of these considerations we adopt the solution that when a uterus is so badly damaged that competent and conscientious obstetricians judge that it has been traumatized beyond a stage where it can be repaired to function safely, they are not obliged to repair it but may remove it, with the consent of the patient.

However, as in so many other matters, the caution not to adopt the "rule of thumb" is indicated here. In view of the history of caesarean sections, it would certainly be impossible to say that a uterus may always be considered functionally dangerously pathological after any previously specified number of sections.

Moreover, since this sacrifice of the generative system can be justified only under the principle of double effect, the required proportion between the good effect and the evil effect must be kept constantly in view. The doctor must always judge the degree of danger inherent in the surgical trauma of these particular scars in this particular uterus. Narvekar has pointed out that the rupture of a caesarean section scar is less of a catastrophe than the rupture of a previously uninjured uterus and that, granted ordinary precautions, the maternal mortality associated with scar rupture is not greater than that associated with routine repeat sections.[104]

This is borne out by Dr. Joseph P. Donnelly's remarks at the 1954 meeting of the New York Obstetrical Society in regard to the fifty-eight uterine ruptures that occurred at the Margaret Hague Hospital between 1931 and 1953.

Dr. Donnelly points out that these fifty-eight ruptures represent one in every 2,662 deliveries; and of the fifty-eight ruptures, seventeen were traumatic, eighteen were spontaneous, and twenty-three occurred in scars of previous caesarean sections; but that while the maternal mortality rate was 21%, no deaths occurred among the ruptures of previous caesarean section scars.[105] These studies are presented by way of balancing the question, and are certainly not meant to imply that scar-rupture is anything less than an extremely serious eventuality.

While theological opinion supports solid probability for hysterectomy in these cases, this is liable to present another moral question which can be phrased as follows: in the case of a patient for whom a procedure so extensive as hysterectomy is surgically contraindicated, would it be morally acceptable to merely isolate the damaged uterus instead of totally removing it from the pelvis?

Hysterectomy after repeated caesarean sections may well be complicated by pelvic and bladder adhesions, usually requires transfusion, and is definitely a major surgical undertaking which, in some cases, may be extremely dangerous at the time of caesarean section.

In the presence of a real clinical exigency, it is my opinion that the isolation procedure would be morally acceptable.[106] It should be noted in this regard that in the process of an indicated hysterectomy, an early part of the surgical technique would consist in the clamping and dividing of the Fallopian tubes in the process of freeing the uterus from its adnexa. When this stage of the surgery has been accomplished, the dangerous uterus has already been effectively isolated from the rest of the system and at this point of the surgery one has already passed through the moral issue involved. Whether the thus effectively isolated uterus is now actually removed from the pelvic cavity, or allowed to remain there, seems to be without moral significance. It can, however, be of extremely important medical significance when the patient is not in a physical condition adequate to withstand the greater impact of the more extensive operation.

Although I believe that this opinion has valid application under the principles of probabilism, experience has clearly demonstrated that there is considerable danger of it being misunderstood and extended far beyond its theological basis. The legitimate concept of "uterine isolation" applies *only* to the instance in which hysterectomy is indicated because of dangerous pathology within the uterus itself (which will obviously be mechanical rather than malignant), and in which the isolation of the uterus would be an acceptable clinical substitute for a morally and clinically defensible hysterectomy.

Unfortunately many physicians, either deviously or through moral ignorance, have latched onto the term "uterine isolation" and semantically substituted it for "tubal ligation" in an attempt to defend direct sterilization. Such semantic distortion, whether by deceit or defect, is unworthy of the profession.

CHAPTER FIVE

MORAL ASPECTS OF PREGNANCY AND DELIVERY

Many of the most common and difficult moral problems which confront the physician arise out of the complications which may be involved in the course of pregnancy, or at the time of delivery.

In the cases under consideration here, the moral problem usually stems from the fact that two human lives, the life of the mother, and the life of the fetus, are in question.

The principle of the inviolability of human life primarily delineates what cannot be done in such a situation. Obviously the destruction of the life of one individual cannot become a mere means to saving the life of the other. This is the most important of the fundamental principles involved in the moral problems of obstetrics.

On the other hand, some of the therapeutic procedures used in the complications of pregnancy, while not directly attacking either the maternal or the fetal life, do result in danger, more or less great, to one or the other. It is in such a situation that the principle of double effect will indicate what can be done.

Perhaps the most common misconception and misunderstanding in the lay mind on this subject, and the one which the Catholic doctor will be called upon most frequently to answer, is the idea that a Catholic doctor, in a difficult obstetrical situation, is obliged to save the child at the expense of the mother's life.

The fact is simply this: There can be no direct attack either on the life of the mother, or on the life of the unborn child. The misunderstanding persists in spite of the fact that pronouncements of the Holy See on the subject have been numerous and constant.

As long ago as November, 1951 Pius XII very clearly stated:

Never and in no case has the Church taught that the life of the child must be preferred to that of the mother. It is erroneous to put the question with this alternative: either the life of the child or that of the mother. No, neither the life of the mother nor that of the child can be subjected to an act of direct suppression. In the one case, as in the other, there can be but one obligation: to make every effort to save the lives of both, of the mother and of the child.[107]

If complications are present during pregnancy or at delivery in which the doctor, in order to save the life either of the mother or of the child, has to institute treatment during the course of which one or the other will perish, or at least be in very serious danger, he may, under these conditions, institute such treatment. But the treatment must be, of its very nature, primarily directed at saving the life either of the mother or of the child, and not directly destructive of the life of either.

To the question: which life is to be preferred?, or which life is to be saved?, there can be no general answer. The dilemma is normally solved by the circumstances of the individual case. In any given case, the nature of the disorder or the trauma determines which one possibly can be saved. But even then, in order to save one, the other cannot be directly destroyed.

The psychological process which keeps this error of the supposed child-mother preference in the Catholic hospital so persistently viable is worthy of brief consideration. In other hospitals which allow therapeutic abortion, the opposite is true—namely, that the life of the mother is preferred to the life of the child. Indeed, in many cases the unborn child is destroyed in the interest of the mother's health, or even in the interest of her psychological comfort. This, of course, represents an erroneous appreciation of the value of intrauterine human life. But error has a way of twisting the truth to conceal itself. The fact is that this indefensible preference for the life and comfort of the mother is denied in a Catholic hospital, where both the maternal and the fetal life are treated with equal reverence, and the inviolability of each is equally respected. The error that in a Catholic hospital the life of the child is preferred to that of the mother is a distortion of fact which tends to persist because, in many other hospitals, the opposite is true.

Abortion

Presupposing a thorough understanding of the principles regarding the inviolability of human life, a medical-moral discussion need not be concerned at great length with the morality of abortion, as that word is commonly understood, since it represents an obvious usurpation of the exclusively divine prerogative of absolute dominion over human life.

There is, however, a real necessity for enucleating very clear concepts of the definition of the term "abortion" in its medical, moral, legal, and canonical use.

Medical Terminology: Medical texts normally give a generic definition of abortion as the termination of a pregnancy, at any time after the fetus has implanted in the uterine wall and before viability.

Since, however, the usual obstetric textbook differentiates abortion from embryotomy (the dismembering and sometimes evisceration of the fetus in utero), craniotomy (the destruction of the fetal head in utero to facilitate the emptying of the uterus), and termination of extopic pregnancy (the removal of a non-viable fetus whose site of gestation is extra-uterine), it seems that the following would be acceptable as a specific breakdown of the medical meaning of the term:

Abortion: The separation of a non-viable fetus from the uterus.

Spontaneous Abortion: Abortion occurring naturally.

Induced Abortion: An abortion which is precipitated artificially and purposely.

Induced abortion is further subdivided into therapeutic abortion and criminal abortion:

Therapeutic Abortion: An abortion induced artificially and purposely, in order to save the life of the mother, or in the interests of the maternal health, or even her mental comfort.

Criminal Abortion: An abortion induced artificially and purposely and in violation of the civil law.

Legal Terminology

The civil law concerns itself primarily with induced abortion, as it differentiates between therapeutic and criminal abortion.

Until well beyond the first half of the present century, the legal aspects of abortion in the United States were determined by the statute law of the various states, generally determining abortion as a felony, unless it was done to preserve the life of the mother or, in a few jurisdictions, also to protect her health. As the medical profession, however, continued to veer further away from the Hippocratic oath, broader indications for abortion were accepted by many physicians, and the courts generally ignored violations of the law, as long as the abortions were performed in a proper clinical setting. In effect, the only practical identification of "criminal abortion" (in the application of the law) was an abortion that was done under cover, either by an unqualified operator or for reasons that few other physicians would publicly endorse. This, of course, was symptomatic of the situational ethic which was rapidly eroding the moral integrity of society.

The situational ethic which necessarily arises from a materialistic and utilitarian philosophy of life falsely tends to make current human conduct, on the part of some, the norm of the natural law rather than discern objective right order as the norm of human conduct. Indeed, such a philosophy of life has little else to draw on and finds itself without any ultimate norm, save the convenience of those who can make themselves heard. It is difficult enough to understand how one can reasonably adopt this attitude toward human life. It is even more difficult to see how it can be done without denying the validity of the very foundations of our democratic way of life enunciated in our own American Declaration of Independence, for it implies a denial of those fundamental and absolute rights and truths, which the founding Fathers held to be self-evident.

This approach to abortion was explicitly legalized twenty years ago in Europe when, in 1946, Sweden greatly broadened its grounds for legal abortion in an attempt to eliminate criminal and septic abortion. But by 1951, Sweden's legal abortion rate had reached 57.4 per 1,000 live births, with no evidence of a decrease in criminal abortions.[108]

In 1955, Soviet Russia legalized abortion at the mere request of the pregnant mother as well as for very broad sociological indications. Most of the Iron Curtain countries quickly followed suit, and by 1959, legal abortion had risen to one tenth of the number of live births in Poland, and to one third of the number of live births in both Bulgaria and Czechoslovakia. In Hungary the number of abortions exceeded the number of live births.[109]

In 1959, the American Law Institute included a section in its Model Penal Code (Section 207.11) which would dramatically expand the legal indications for abortion in the United States, so as to include substantial risk to the mental health of the mother, or the risk that the child would be born with grave physical or mental defect, or in the event that the pregnancy resulted from rape or incest. Organized pressure was brought to bear on various state legislatures to adopt this type of code, such as was organized in Kansas in 1963, in New York in 1964, and in California in 1965.

Finally, the Supreme Court of the United States, in its landmark decisions of 1971 (*Roe vs. Wade—Doe vs. Bolton*) created the legal framework for abortion-on-demand in the United States. The court ruled that in the first trimester of pregnancy, the abortion decision must be left to the medical judgment of the physician, and that in the second trimester "the State, in promoting its interest in the health of the mother, may, if it chooses, regulate the abortion procedure in ways that are reasonably related to maternal health." (*Roe vs. Wade*, pp. 43-44). The Court further in medically anomalous terms said that after viability, the State could "regulate and even proscribe abortion except where it is necessary, in appropriate medical judgment, for the preservation of the life or health of the mother." (*Roe vs. Wade*, pp. 44-48). The medical anomaly lies on the fact that termination of pregnancy after viability, although dangerous to the survival of the baby in proportion to the anticipation of term, is not abortion at all, but is rather referred to as premature delivery.

Moral Terminology: The moral theologian is concerned with abortion in its relation to the inviolability of human life. The moralist thus recognizes the medical distinction between spontaneous and induced abortion, but in the latter category fails to perceive any valid distinction between therapeutic and criminal abortion. Moreover, it is to be noted that the moral concept does not limit the idea of abortion to the period subsequent to implantation in the uterine wall (as does the usual medical understanding of the term), but considers any destruction of the products of human conception as an abortion, whether before or after implantation. This concept is particularly germane to the moral evaluation of those intrauterine devices and "contraception" medications which may prevent implantation rather than conception.

The moral theologians do, however, introduce a new set of terminology by their use of the terms: "direct" and "indirect" abortion.

Direct Abortion: A direct abortion is one which is intended either as an end in itself, or as a means to an end. Since, in such a case, the procedure of emptying the uterus is precisely and directly intended for the purpose of interrupting the pregnancy, it clearly constitutes a direct attack on the life of the non-viable fetus.

Indirect Abortion: Uterine evacuation of a non-viable fetus which is foreseen but merely permitted, i.e., not the intended or directly willed result of, but the side-effect of, a procedure which is directed toward some good end and legitimate purpose, is called indirect abortion.

Canonical Terminology: The canonist uses the terms in the same sense as does the moral theologian, being particularly careful, however, to classify abortion as the separation of a non-viable *living* fetus from the *uterus*, thus sharply distinguishing abortion, in its canonical concept, from craniotomy and embryotomy.

The reason for this distinction is that in inflicting of ecclesiastical penalties, the law is to be interpreted strictly, i.e., the words of the law are to be understood according to the meaning which would narrow, rather than enlarge, the application of the penalty.[110] As will be seen later, canon law on abortion deals with the penalty of excommunication.

Coordination of Terminology:

1. The specific definition of abortion as the separation of a living non-viable fetus from the uterus, and the distinction between induced and spontaneous abortion, would be acceptable to the obstetrician, the lawyer, the moralist, and the canonist alike.

2. The medico-legal distinction between therapeutic and criminal abortion is repudiated by the moralist and canonist. The theologians would classify both of these as direct abortion.

3. The more evident distinction between the medical spontaneous and induced abortion is based on the ideas of "natural" and "artificially induced." However, because induced abortion also contains the note "of set purpose," we believe that the moral term "indirect abortion" should be associated with the medical "spontaneous." Even though the uterine evacuation of indirect abortion is the result of some artificial procedure, in the moral order this artificial procedure has no direct connection with the uterine evacuation. The indirect abortion is properly described as the spontaneous result of an artificially produced condition in the mother.

Moral Aspects of Abortion

Direct abortion, whether it be classified as therapeutic abortion or criminal abortion, is always and under all circumstances in direct violation of the natural law and the divine positive law.

It is the usurpation of the uniquely divine prerogative of absolute dominion over human life.

From the Council of Elvira (*circa* A.D. 300) to Vatican II the Catholic Church has always condemned abortion of the human fetus as the murder of the innocent. Even during those periods of Church History, particularly from the twelfth to the nineteenth century, when the more severe canonical penalties for abortion were based on the medically popular delayed animation theories of the time, still severe penalties were sometimes inflicted for abortion, which was done even before the supposed animation of the fetus; and sometimes such abortions were referred to as "conditional" or "interpretive" homicide. It is, of course, true that those who accepted the delayed animation theory as certain, did not identify abortion before the fetus was considered human as simple murder. But, as will be pointed out later, the collapse of the general acceptability of the delayed animation theory in modern medicine leaves this without relevance today.[111]

This does not mean that no moral theologians, in the history of the Church, have ever speculated about, or individually sought to defend, the liceity of abortion under some extreme circumstances. As mentioned above, some held that very early abortion was permissible under the delayed animation theory, when this was a commonly accepted medical premise, and some few even sought to defend late abortion under the principle of the unjust aggressor, or as the lesser of two evils, or as a necessity for baptizing the fetus, or even under the presumed willingness of the child to sacrifice its right to life for the safety of its mother. But all of these theories were shown to be erroneous and deficient, and in the history of Catholic thinking they were never accepted by the Church as Catholic doctrine.[112]

The delayed animation theory merits some comment. The philosophical-physiological-theological speculations as to when the products of human conception are human (i.e., endowed with an individual soul or principle of independent human life, albeit still within the womb and physically dependent on the mother) has never been, and perhaps never will be, definitively settled. But whether the new and distinct human life is present from the moment of conception, or at some later stage of gestation is not greatly significant, because the malice of abortion lies in the willingness to destroy intra-uterine life, although it is human or, in the very earliest stages of gestation, *even if* it is human. Hippocrates, Aristotle and Galen, all struggled with the problem of the moment of specifically human animation, as did Tertullian and Apollinaris, Basil and Gregory of Nissa, Jerome and Augustine, and Thomas Aquinas. The most common theory, that the conceptus passed through a vegetative and animal stage, finally becoming human at about the fortieth day in the case of males and the eightieth day in the case of females, is by no means bizarre against the background of the scientific method of the times. Men have generally concluded that things are probably what they appear to be. To the naked eye, a conceptus in its early stages does look like a sea anemone, and by the time an embryo is observable, it looks like any animal embryo. At about forty days the phallic tubercule makes every embryo look more like a human male than a female, and the external genitalia of the female are not clearly discernible to the naked eye until about the eightieth day. And with the theory accepted medically, it is not surprising that some theologians thought they saw confirmatory references in the Book of Leviticus (12:2-5) where the purification period of the parturient similarly varies according to the sex of the child.

While the moment of new human life still evades any known investigative process, it is interesting to note that the same scientific method of observation, aided today by modern microscopy, indicates chromosomal patterns in the nuclei of the earliest stages of cell division as specifically human, and indeed personally individualized already, thus seeming to support the probability that, from the moment of conception, John is John, and not George.[113]

At any rate, the only practical working premise is to treat the human conceptus as if the moment of a new and distinct human life were certainly the moment of conception, as the Code of Canon Law does with regard to Baptism (canon 747) and abortion (canon 2350). Since the soul may very likely be present from that moment, to directly destroy the products of human conception, even at a very early stage of development, is at least very likely the destruction of an innocent human life. One who does even this, has already discarded, from his moral code, the inviolability of human life, and falls far short of that regard for the dignity and rights of the individual, which is basic to the entire Judaico-Christian theology and tradition, as well as to the American way of life. Such an action is at least identified with the moral malice of murder, since it implies a willingness to kill, even if human life is there.

As early as the fourth century, St. Basil pointed out exactly the same analysis of the malice of abortion and wrote, regarding the fetus: "any fine distinction as to its being completely formed or informed is not admissible among us," and he referred to those who give drugs to procure abortion, and to those who take them, as "murderers."[114]

Likewise, in our own time, Pius XI, Pius XII and John XXIII have condemned abortion in very similar terms; as has Pope Paul VI:

Pius XI: As to the 'medical and therapeutic indication' to which, using their own words, we have made reference, Venerable Brethren, however much we may pity the mother whose health and even life is gravely imperiled in the performance of the duty allotted to her by nature, nevertheless, what could ever be a sufficient reason for excusing in any way the direct murder of the innocent? This is precisely what we are dealing with here.[115]

Pius XII: Innocent human life, in whatever condition it is found, is withdrawn, from the very first moment of its existence, from any direct deliberate attack. This is a fundamental right of the human person, which is of general value in the Christian concept of life; hence as valid for the life still hidden within the womb of the mother, as for the life already born and developing outside of her, as much opposed to direct abortion as to the direct killing of the child before, during, or after its birth. Whatever foundation there may be for the distinction between these various phases of the development of life that is born, or still unborn, in profane and ecclesiastical law, and as regards certain civil and penal consequences, all these cases involve a grave and unlawful attack upon the inviolability of human life.[116]

John XXIII: Human life is sacred—all men must recognize that fact. From its very inception, it reveals the creating hand of God. Those who violate His laws not only offend the divine majesty and degrade themselves and humanity, they also sap the vitality of the political community of which they are members.[117]

Paul VI: We are certain that the consciousness of your professional function will illuminate and guide your skillful medical art, and that, in the exercise of your practice, you will always recall the principles of ethics, which Christian morals raise to their highest and most exigent expression, particularly when it is a matter of defending the life of each human being. You know that the voice of the Church, acting as interpreter of that Christian law, was heard in the teaching of Our Predecessor, Pope Pius XII, concerning a fundamental point, when he said: 'Innocent human life, in whatever condition it is found, is withdrawn, from the very first moment of its existence, from any direct deliberate attack. . .'.[118]

Even more recently, on November 18, 1974, the Vatican Congregation for the Doctrine of the Faith issued a lengthy declaration, ratified and confirmed by Pope Paul VI, reviewing and reaffirming Catholic teaching on abortion.

Indirect abortion involves certain moral problems, many of which are treated in some detail in the following pages. Moral questions regarding indirect abortion will usually be solved under the principle of double effect.

Abortion and the Code of Canon Law

Here it is of paramount importance to recognize the difference between Moral Theology and Canon Law, as well as their proper mutual relationships. The Church in the world is described as a saving presence, as the people of God, formed by the Will of Christ and fashioned by His Holy Spirit, in a function of service and mission achieved primarily through its own sanctification, its union with Christ. Theology is both the discernment of Christ's revelation (Dogmatic Theology) and the application of that revelation to human conduct (Moral Theology). But as an externally visible society, the Church has an internal government charged with the right ordering of the ecclesial society itself (Canon Law).

Good government involves laws, and laws beget an appropriate legalism. Indeed, in civil society the entire juridical system attests to this fact. Legal penalties, whether ecclesiastical or civil, should be clearly defined, concisely understood and (as is explicitly noted in the Code of Canon Law), stringently restricted in their scope. Thus, there is a necessary and appropriate difference between the charism of theology and the interpretative legalism of Canon Law.

The following notations, without being a comprehensive treatment of the many ramifications and details of ecclesiastical penalties, should supply an adequate understanding of the salient features of the canonical excommunication attached to the crime of direct abortion.

We will first quote, in part, canon 2350 of the Code of Canon Law, and then attempt to clarify this legislation by a closer examination of the wording of the law itself:

Canon 2350: "Those who procure abortion, not excepting the mother, incur, if the effect is produced, an excommunication *latae sententiae* reserved to the Ordinary..."

Abortion: The technical interpretation of the word "abortion" in the Code of Canon Law immediately presents a valid canonical-legal distinction. Penalties are to be interpreted restrictively (Canon 19) and the narrowest medical understanding of "abortion" is "the separation of a living non-viable fetus (or embryo) from the uterus." Therefore neither prevention of implantation, nor craniotomy, embryotomy, nor the illicit removal of a ectopic fetus, whether tubal, ovarian, or abdominal, although equally serious crimes, are punished by this ecclesiastical penalty.

Procure: Means by direct intention, or what has been described as direct abortion.

Not excepting the mother: These words simply clarify a pre-code dispute as to whether or not the mother was subject to this ecclesiastical penalty.

If the effect is produced: To incur the penalty, it does not suffice that an act designed to cause abortion has been performed, but it must likewise be clear that the abortion has occurred, and occurred as a result of this act.

Moreover, when the words: "If the effect is produced" are found in the law, canonists discuss whether or not the censure is incurred, if repentance ensues between the time that the criminal action takes place, and the time that the effect (abortion in this case) actually occurs. The question is pertinent to the present matter, since this time lapse could be considerable in some cases of abortion. Although canonists disagree on the question, their very disagreement would render the censure doubtful if repentance ensues before the abortion actually occurs. Since the Code of Canon Law lays down the principle of benign interpretation of penal law, the milder opinion is to be followed in practice.[119]

Excommunication: A popular misunderstanding in the lay mind with regard to excommunication is that if excommunication is incurred, the excommunicated individual is "out of the Church." This is false. An excommunication is an ecclesiastical penalty, which deprives one of the right to assist at divine services, to receive the sacraments, and to share in the indulgences and public prayers of the Church. It is effective until absolved. However, it is false to say that in virtue of excommunication one ceases to be a Catholic, or is relieved of his obligations as a Catholic.

Latae sententiae: This is a technical canonical term which means that the excommunication is incurred automatically, once the crime has been committed.

Reserved to the Ordinary: This means that only the bishop of the diocese, or someone with special faculties from him, or from the Roman Pontiff, can absolve the excommunication.

Additional Notations about Excommunication: In order for a canonical penalty of this nature to be effective, there must be certainty that the crime was committed, that it fulfills the definition of the crime in the law, and that the culprit was acting with the sufficient knowledge and consent required for serious sin.

Moreover, it is necessary that the culprit, at the time that he committed the crime, knew that such a crime was punished by some ecclesiastical penalty.

Moreover, if one committed this crime under the pressure of grave fear, even though he might sin mortally, he would not incur the excommunication.

Canonical Principles of Cooperation: Previously, we have dealt with the *"moral* principles of cooperation." It is extremely important to note here that these are not exactly the same as the *"canonical* principles of cooperation." The concept of cooperation in canon law is a juridical concept. The law does not concern itself primarily with an investigation into which types of cooperation are sinful and which are not, but rather with the question of which types of cooperation are, by positive legislation, punished by an ecclesiastical penalty. Hence the canonist's approach to the problem is slightly different from that of the moralist.

Cooperation in a crime is had when there is the participation of more than one person in the same crime.

We have seen that the ecclesiastical penalty of excommunication is inflicted upon one who performs an abortion. The same penalty is also incurred by some of those who actually assist in the commission of the crime.

The mere intention to assist at an abortion could certainly be seriously sinful. But to incur the excommunication, one must *actually assist,* either physically or morally. It must constantly be remembered, in dealing with this matter, that we are dealing with the *canonical,* and not the moral, concept of cooperation.

Cooperation in a crime can be *physical* (by actually physically helping someone to commit a crime) or *moral* (by encouragement, persuasion, etc.).

Cooperation in a crime can be *physically necessary* (if the crime, de facto, *could not* have been committed without such cooperation) or physically *non-necessary* (if the crime could have been committed without such cooperation).

Whether *moral cooperation* is *necessary* or *non-necessary* depends on whether or not the crime *would have been* committed without such cooperation.

Cooperation in a crime can be *"with previous agreement"* (as when two or more people mutually agree to assist in what they know to be a crime), or *"without previous agreement"* (as when someone just happens to be present and assists in the crime).

Cooperation can be *"in the acts preparatory to the crime,"* or *"in the acts which initiate the crime,"* or *"during the commission of the crime."*

Canon 2209 outlines the salient features of canonical cooperation in a crime to which a canonical penalty is attached. It reads, in part, as follows:

Canon 2209/1: "Persons who conspire to commit a crime and physically concur in it are all held equally guilty, unless circumstances increase or diminish the guilt of some or one of them."

Canon 2209/3: "Not only the one who commits a crime and is thus the principal culprit, but also those who induce the commission of the crime, or concur in it in any way, incur no less guilt, other things being equal, than the one who perpetrated it, if without their help the crime would not have been committed."

Hence, regarding the crime of abortion:

1. Those who physically concur in the actual abortion, either by explicit, or at least implicit previous agreement, or without previous agreement, but as necessary cooperators, incur the penalty of excommunication. This would include everyone actually engaged in the operating room, either by previous agreement or as necessary agents, from the moment the operation actually begins until the abortion is complete.

2. Those who, with or without previous agreement, concur physically by acts preparatory to the abortion, or in the initial acts of the abortion, or during the abortion itself, incur the censure if the abortion could not have been performed without their cooperation.

Preparation acts: e.g., preparation of the operating room, preparation of the patient on the ward, transfer of the patient from ward bed to operating theatre, etc.

Initial acts: e.g., preparation of sterile field on body of patient, beginning anesthesia, etc.

During the abortion: e.g., anesthesia after surgery is begun, holding retractors, passing instruments, etc.

3. Those who order, encourage, or persuade abortion incur the censure, if the abortion would not have been performed without their moral cooperation.

4. Others, at an administrative level, who could and should prevent the abortion, and *agree* not to do so, likewise incur the penalty of excommunication.

Examples of Canonical Cooperation

All other things being equal (supposing subjective knowledge required for serious sin, awareness of penalty, etc.), the following individuals would incur the excommunication as cooperators in abortion:

1. A Catholic doctor tells his patient that, with her cardiac complication, she should have her pregnancy terminated by means of a therapeutic abortion. He explains that, as a Catholic, he cannot do this himself, but refers her to another member of the staff who will do it, and the woman does have the abortion.

The doctor is a necessary moral cooperator. It was he who determined the woman's will to have the abortion.

2. A medical student is present when a surgeon asks for someone to scrub in on a therapeutic abortion. He volunteers his services. During the operation all he does is hold the retractors.

The medical student is physically cooperating during the actual abortion, and even though he is a non-necessary cooperator (because the surgeon could have engaged someone else), he is, nonetheless, cooperating "by previous agreement."

3. The only hospital available has a policy contrary to therapeutic abortion. The admitting officer of this hospital

knows that a woman is coming to the hospital in order to have a therapeutic abortion. When her doctor applies for a room, he assigns one, which he could legitimately refuse to do.

The admitting officer is a necessary physical cooperator in an act preparatory to the abortion.

The following cooperators would not incur the excommunication:

1. In case number 3 above, the chief of surgery knows that a doctor in his department is going to perform the abortion. The chief does not stop him because he is reluctant to enter into this problem. He just ignores the whole situation and says nothing. Although the chief has a duty to prevent the abortion, his cooperation is strictly negative and negligent. There is no previous agreement, either explicit or implicit, with the abortionist. Thus although his negligence is seriously wrong and irresponsible, he technically does not incur the censure.

2. The regular anesthetist, while administering anesthetic during a laparotomy, notices that the surgeon is performing an abortion. The anesthetist continues to administer the anesthetic.

Although cooperating during the abortion itself, this particular anesthetist is presumed not to be a necessary cooperator. His cooperation is evidently without previous agreement.

3. The chief resident in anesthesiology sees a therapeutic abortion scheduled, to which he is assigned for anesthesia. He disapproves, but knows that if he refuses to be present or makes an issue of it, he will lose his residency and endanger his career. The surgeon asks him if he will administer the anesthetic, and he says that he will. He had consulted the hospital chaplain who told him that under these circumstances, in the light of the principles of moral cooperation, it would not be sinful for him to administer the anesthetic.

Even though the chief resident is cooperating during the actual abortion, and in a sense, by previous agreement, his action is, under the particular circumstances, not sinful. Therefore, he cannot incur the penalty.

Medical Aspects of Abortion

Obstetrics has witnessed an interesting but tragic revolution in the twentieth century. In the early years of this century the textbooks listed many medical indications for therapeutic abortion in the interest of the maternal life. As obstetric research and improved technique reduced the medical indications for abortion to near zero, the discouraging fact remained that many pregnant mothers simply did not want to give birth to their babies. Thus there was a long period in which obsolete medical indications became medical excuses rather than reasons for aborting. Finally, while the civil law still required a medical indication if abortion was to be done, there was a shift to nebulous and unproven psychiatric indications and to the unusual concept of abortion in the interest of the unborn baby under the questionable presupposition of "better dead than deaf" (the rubella rubric) or "better dead than disdained" (the unwanted baby warranty).

Subsequent to the decision of the Supreme Court to abandon protection of the unborn, reasons for aborting are seldom required. Where a reason is given, it is often medically obsolete or psychiatrically unfounded.

It might be noted that the relevance of much that follows here is not limited to the question of abortion, but is obviously likewise related to those many instances in which some physicians call for contraceptive sterilization because, as they say (too often, not without exaggeration), another pregnancy would mean death for the mother.

The medical trend away from abortion (subsequent to the advent of modern obstetric technique and prior to the current legalized abortion craze), was well summed up in the words of Dr. Roy J. Heffernan, of Tufts Medical College, as reported in the San Francisco press on the occasion of a symposium on therapeutic abortion at the 1951 meeting of The American College of Surgeons. Dr. Heffernan said, on that occasion: "Anyone who performs a therapeutic abortion is either ignorant of modern medical methods, or unwilling to take the time and effort to apply them."[120]

For example, although in an earlier survey on therapeutic abortion, one hospital was reported to have one therapeutic abortion for every thirty-five obstetrical admissions, the Margaret Hague Maternity Hospital in Jersey City reported a ratio of less than one therapeutic abortion in every sixteen thousand admissions.

Dr. Frederick L. Good, as Surgeon-in-Chief of Boston City Hospital's Obstetric and Gynecological Service, reported in March 1951, that there had been no therapeutic abortion in that hospital since March 1, 1923, and that during that time the mortality rate due to conditions supposedly benefited by therapeutic abortion had been zero.[121]

Moreover, Dr. Heffernan and Dr. William A. Lynch, basing their remarks on a study of over three million deliveries, reported the following interesting fact in the literature:

> Of special interest is the fact that the maternal mortality rates in the hospitals performing therapeutic abortions, while excellent, were not better than those in the hospitals wherein no therapeutic abortions were performed. In fact, a few more mothers died in the hospitals allowing therapeutic abortions.[122]

In the summary and conclusions of the same article, these two well-known obstetricians make the following significant observations:

> As therapeutic abortion involves the direct destruction of human life, it is contrary to all the rules and traditions of good medical practice. From the very beginning, the approach to the problem has been unscientific. In too many cases it was learned, after innumerable babies had been sacrificed, that interruption of the pregnancy not only caused 100 per cent fetal loss, but also increased the maternal mortality.

Craniotomy

In the broadest sense of the word, any operation on the skull is properly referred to as craniotomy. However, the term is normally used in an obstetrical reference to indicate the opening of the fetal head and the evacuation of the skull content, followed by a reduction of the size of the head by means of crushing the skull, so that the fetal head can be more easily delivered through the parturient canal. Note the following quotations from obstetrical texts:

Titus: The commonest indication for craniotomy is hydrocephalus. Hydrocephalus of sufficient degree to cause disproportion and dystocia is certain to produce idiocy in the child, so that there is no excuse, either sentimental or otherwise, for making the mother undergo the risk of a caesarean section in order to deliver an hydrocephalic child alive. Craniotomy is indicated whether the infant is alive or dead.

In the presence of hydrocephalus, craniotomy on the living infant will be refused by the family if they are Catholic. O'Connor and Gorman recommend for this situation that intraventricular tap and drainage be accomplished by means of a trochar passed through the cervical canal. This usually diminishes the head sufficiently to allow it to be born without dystocia or mutilation, and being identical with the familiar therapeutic drainage of an hydrocephalic child in infancy, objection is not offered to it by the Catholic Church.[123]

Eastman: It (craniotomy) is never employed today on living infants, except in cases of hydrocephalus... In this condition a destructive operation is more readily undertaken, as even a successful caesarean section will only give us a child that is doomed to die shortly or to remain an idiot. If, in the case of hydrocephalus, there are religious objections to the usual form of craniotomy, a spinal puncture needle may be inserted through the most accessible suture space and sufficient fluid withdrawn to allow descent of the head through the pelvis. In the few cases in which I have done this, delivery has been prompt, and there have been no discernible effects of a harmful nature on the infant, but of course the hydrocephalic condition develops again subsequently.[124]

Moral Aspects: It seems unnecessary to repeat again the obvious fact that no man, on his own authority or on any but divine authority, is ever justified in directly killing another human being.

Certainly we cannot agree with those obstetrical writers who say that, since the child is going to be born an idiot, or die soon anyhow, there is no excuse, "either sentimental or otherwise," for subjecting the mother to the risk of a caesarean section; no more than we could agree that since everyone is going to die eventually, murder of the unfortunate is perfectly all right; as long as it benefits some third party. Note the following comment of Cunningham:

> No obstetrician, worthy of the name, would perform such an operation (craniotomy) on a living fetus. In cases of obstructed delivery from any cause, it is always possible to effect the safe delivery of the fetus by some operative method, without undue risk to the mother. This is especially true at the present time, when operative procedures have been brought to such a high stage of perfection and when there is recourse to potent anti-bacterial agents.[125]

It is to be noted, however, that mutilating operations of the fetus such as the removal of an arm or leg, or even cranial operations which are not necessarily death-dealing but are an attempt to salvage a trapped fetus, are permitted as a last resort, even though they are very dangerous to the life of the fetus.

The parts of the body, as parts, do exist for the good of the whole; and the removal or mutilation of them in an attempt to salvage the whole is perfectly in accord with right order.

Cleidotomy

It seems advisable to make some explicit mention of cleidotomy, which is described as the surgical procedure of unilateral or bilateral division of the baby's clavicles, in a difficult delivery, in order to permit passage of the shoulders. This operation is sometimes employed when this particular dystocia is discovered only after the head has come forth.

Cleidotomy merits particular attention, because it was normally treated in the obstetric texts under the heading of those operations which are "destructive of the fetus." Of a dozen texts consulted, only three related the operation to a life-saving procedure. The others treated it exclusively as a destructive operation, or at least referred to cleidotomy only in relation to a dead fetus.

In view of the following passages from competent obstetrical texts, it is evident that cleidotomy (cutting the clavicles) or osteoclasis (fracture of the clavicles), is permitted when such a procedure is necessary in an attempt to save the life of the child.

> *Davis and Carter:* The procedure (cleidotomy) was originally intended for use only on a dead fetus, but a few operators have employed it as a life-saving measure when the shoulders are so broad that a delivery cannot be completed after the head has been born.[126]
>
> *Titus:* This operation (cleidotomy) consists of dividing the clavicles in order to collapse a shoulder girdle, the girth of which is so great that the infant cannot be extracted although the head has been born... Both clavicles are divided. This is not necessarily a fatal type of embryotomy nor mutilating beyond recovery.[127]

Addison's Disease

The inadequate function of the suprarenal glands is viewed as the primary disorder of Addison's Disease. The symptoms of severe prostration, progressive anemia, low blood pressure, diarrhea and digestive disturbances have yielded markedly, however, to the advent of the adrenocortical steroids. Part of the result of this possibility of amelioration is that, although previously pregnancy and delivery were viewed as serious risks in the presence of Addison's Disease, the modern obstetrician is not so willing to view the situation with such alarm. The medical literature sounds a much more hopeful note, pointing out that special precautions are necessary, but are now readily available; and that the prognosis of pregnancy in the presence of Addison's Disease is quite favorable.[128] Therapeutic abortion is morally unacceptable.

Cancer of the Breast

Cancer of the breast coexisting with pregnancy is considered by some physicians to be an indication for immediate therapeutic abortion. This judgment is based on the consideration that the increased hormone activity of pregnancy is likely to have a deleterious effect on the growth and spread of the breast cancer, lighting up cells which may be inhibited or inactive, and that the termination of pregnancy spells the reduction of this hormone activity.

Breast cancer is a formidable and frequently fatal disease. Yet, as Pope Pius XI wrote in the encyclical already quoted:

> However much we may pity the mother whose health and even life is gravely imperiled in the performance of the duty allotted to her by nature, nevertheless what could ever be a sufficient reason for excusing in any way the direct murder of the innocent? This is precisely what we are dealing with here.[129]

Moreover, the theory which is proposed as a clinical defense of this direct destruction of fetal life seems to be, at the very least, highly questionable in its effects. At the meeting of the Central Association of Obstetricians and Gynecologists (Kansas City, Missouri, October 6-8, 1960) Thaddeus Montgomery of Jefferson Medical College reviewed the work of the Committee on Breast Cancer of the Philadelphia Medical Society and advocated therapeutic abortion. He said that:

> In view of the extremely serious nature of carcinoma of the breast, and the profound effect which the enhanced circulation and the stimulus of hormones have upon growth of the lesion, we feel that pregnancy should be promptly terminated. If the patient is within the period of viability, a living fetus may be salvaged. If not, the embryo is sacrificed.[130]

But in the question period following his address, when Dr. Montgomery was asked: "Do you have any statistical evidence that interruption of pregnancy increases the longevity of a woman with cancer of the breast?" his reply was: "No, I haven't and don't know of any sound evidence."

Moreover, many others who are qualified to make sound

clinical judgments would approve breast surgery when necessary and with proper safeguards for the fetus, but would not approve therapeutic abortion. In one published survey of the opinions of fifty-five surgeons in this matter, of the thirty-five who responded to the questionnaire eleven felt that carcinoma of the breast at anytime during pregnancy was an indication for therapeutic abortion and ten felt that there was no reason to abort the fetus. Others were divided regarding the first or second trimester.[131]

Robert Brown, while approving therapeutic abortion in such cases "under certain circumstances and upon theoretical grounds," reported on his own series of cases in the Los Angeles area, and reviewed the world literature on cancer of the breast during pregnancy with the following conclusion:

> Neither interrupting the pregnancy nor allowing it to go to term has affected the ultimate outcome of any patient who has had cancer of the breast. Whether interruption of the pregnancy adds to the patient's lifetime cannot be determined from this study or from available information of the world literature.[132]

Holleb and Farrow, after a study of 283 cases in New York (at the Memorial Hospital for Cancer and the James Ewing Hospital) over a period of thirty-five years, could find no proof that the interruption of pregnancy increased the survival time of the mother.[133]

The group at Vanderbilt reached essentially the same conclusion in their series: that radical surgery, when indicated for breast cancer, need not be postponed because of pregnancy and that, with proper adjunctive care, pregnancy need not be terminated.[134]

In summary, from a moral viewpoint, if radical mastectomy is urgently indicated during pregnancy, the operation need not be postponed because of danger to the unborn fetus, but therapeutic abortion in these, as in all other circumstances, is indefensible. And even from a strictly medical point of view the observation of Bunker and Peters of the Ontario Cancer Institute is significant. Reviewing their series of 150 cases, they observe

that: "In this group, at least, therapeutic abortion has little beneficial effect. The fetal wastage does not justify the adult salvage."[135]

Cancer of the Cervix

The following consideration, now commonly reported in the
literature, sets the background for considering some of the
moral problems posed by cancer of the cervix during pregnancy.
In contrast to earlier practice, cytology tests during pregnancy
have become routine in many clinics, and the ability to accurately diagnose and distinguish the evidence which indicates
cancer from benign histologic changes in the cervix is more
refined. Questionable laboratory findings are followed up by
punch-biopsy or preferable ring-biopsy (cold-knife conization).
Some of these procedures are not without danger to the pregnancy, depending upon the condition of the patient and the
skill of the operator; but, from a moral viewpoint, the risk
involved here would be considered proportionate to the need
for accurate diagnosis.

After the diagnosis has been made the moral problems increase. Aside from the question of selecting the best elements
for the therapeutic regimen, which will differ according to the
diagnosis of pre-invasive carcinoma in situ or the presence of
already invasive lesions, the consideration of simply doing a
therapeutic abortion arises in some clinics. While direct therapeutic abortion would never be morally acceptable in the context of the Catholic ethic, it would likewise seem to be obstetrically outmoded in cases of carcinoma in situ. Ernest Ayre of
the Cancer Cytology Foundation of America and Joseph Scott
of The University of Miami observe that:

> In the absence of signs of infiltration in repeated cell
> scrapings and histologic studies by cold-knife conization,
> the pregnancy may be allowed to progress to parturition,
> with repeated cell scrapings observed at monthly intervals.
> The treatment of the lesion is to be administered at a suitable
> time after delivery.[136]

Yet, even in this case, if the clinical judgment of the individual surgeon called for direct operative interference on the area of the lesion itself (as distinct from direct therapeutic abortion), even with concomitant loss of the fetus, the moral theologian would respect his judgment. If that judgment were clinically questionable, he would have to defend it to his peers, but not to theologians whose only task is to explain the moral principles involved, and not to make individual applications which involve clinical evaluations.

Ayre and Scott, when dealing with invasive carcinoma, simply state in the same study: "Radical treatment is justified if or when the lesion is found to be clinical and truly invasive or infiltrating." Again, from a moral viewpoint, no one would object to that clinical judgment, but one must take exception to the proposed treatment plan of Stone, Weingold and Small of New York Medical College who, in addition to radical surgery, include direct abortion for its own sake, i.e., to prevent delivery of an abnormal baby presumably compromised by the effects of radiation therapy in the second trimester,[137] nor could one accept the view of Kinch of Western Ontario who simply states that: "In early pregnancy, the patient in the late stages should be treated by x-ray or cobalt beam therapy to produce abortion, followed by radium application to make up the cancercidal dose."[138]

In summary, it may be said that cancer of the cervix during pregnancy, in its various grades and stages, presents highly debatable clinical concepts in both diagnosis and treatment. The theologian can only leave the relative merits of disputed points to the clinician and merely point out that, while the fetus may understandably be lost in the vigorous approach to the lesion, the directly intended abortion of a non-viable, living, albeit hopeless, fetus is viewed as the immoral killing of the innocent.

Cancer of the Rectum

In 1962 O'Leary and Bepko of Georgetown made a review of the principal literature on cancer of the rectum as a complication of pregnancy, documenting the earlier tendency to do therapeutic abortion in these cases. They likewise reviewed the best known successful cases reported in which colostomy was done for obstruction and/or surgery was done for the cancer without disturbance of the pregnancy. Their conclusion is morally sound:

> In cases where the lesion is inoperable . . . the fetus becomes of prime importance, as in our case, and the pregnancy should be allowed to proceed until viability of the fetus seems assured. A colostomy should be done for obstruction. Where the lesion is still operable, one must consider the period of gestation. The generally accepted opinion, where the lesion is discovered during the first or second trimester, is to treat the lesion and disregard the pregnancy.[139]

Moreover, they report, with approval, Warren's conclusion that pregnancy does not adversely affect the course of cancer of the rectum, and that there is no indication for therapeutic abortion.[140]

In such a regimen the operative interference in the first or second trimester is directed solely at the cancerous lesion, and if the fetus should be lost (as may happen in some cases) the abortion is beyond the intention of the surgeon, and, from a moral viewpoint, would be an indirect abortion under the principle of double effect. Third trimester diagnosis suggests a reasonable delay for greater assurance of fetal safety, insofar as this would be in proportion to the maternal welfare.

This is quite different from the suggestion of some: that abortion should be performed first, followed by extensive surgery.[141] Such an approach would be morally unacceptable, as a direct and immediately intended destruction of fetal life.

Cardiac Disease

No one would deny that cardiac disease complicated by pregnancy can sometimes present a delicate and serious clinical crisis. Moreover, it should be evident that a treatise on Medical Ethics is not meant to pose as a therapeutic manual in any sense. What Catholic Theology has to offer might appear to be quite negative from a clinical point of view. It merely states that, even in the presence of severe cardiac complications, the sterilization-abortion approach to pregnancy is not morally acceptable. In a very true sense it is not at all negative, because those physicians who have adhered to it—in the presence of cardiac disease as well as the other complications of pregnancy—have pushed back the frontiers of medicine to advance their art and science, and to save many more lives.

As early as 1943 Gorenberg, while particularly interested in rheumatic heart disease and pregnancy, wrote: "It is probable that practically every pregnancy encountered in a patient with heart disease can be brought to successful spontaneous termination, if adequate prenatal care is instituted, and if absolute bed rest is enforced when indicated."[142] And O'Driscoll, Coyle and Drury of Dublin maintain that therapeutic abortion contributes to neither the immediate nor future welfare of mothers with rheumatic heart disease.[143]

In the 1957 Billings Lecture, Dr. C. Sidney Burwell of the Harvard Medical Faculty referred to the idea that women with heart disease cannot safely have babies as "medical folklore." Reporting on 355 pregnancies in the presence of cardiac disease, Dr. Burwell said:

This total experience indicates to us that in the vast majority of instances, it is possible to carry women with heart disease safely and productively through pregnancy. Success in this endeavor depends on the understanding and careful application of the principle of the total cardiac burden and on making a wide appraisal of the factors, in pregnancy and in other aspects of the patient's life, which influence this burden.[144]

Mitral stenosis has widely been regarded by some clinicians as a definite indication for therapeutic abortion, yet in 1958 William Winter reported that:

Therapeutic abortion as a means of terminating a pregnancy on the basis of mitral stenosis is rapidly becoming an obsolete method of management as a result of the successful utilization of mitral commissurotomy in indicated cases and good conservative management in the remainder.[145]

More recently Burt and Bowden of Bowman Gray noted:

Although the indications for cardiac surgery in relation

to pregnancy remain somewhat controversial, these new techniques have necessarily changed obstetric concepts in many clinics concerning the place of abortion and/or sterilization in the management of the pregnant patient with heart disease.[146]

Again it must be emphasized that these quotations from the literature are obviously not presented here as clinical directives. That would be clearly beyond both the scope and competence of this text. They are presented as almost random examples of current positive thinking, and similar examples can easily be found in relation to the other cardiac complications of pregnancy. And all of this becomes even more deeply significant when viewed against the background of recent legislation which unfortunately has made abortion legally respectable. Is it that the advancing science and art of the medical profession, even as it approaches its peak of excellence, is ready to succumb somewhat to a certain atheistic materialism which has already notably influenced the latter half of the twentieth century? The question is a valid one.

Eclampsia

Eclampsia is described as a toxic disturbance of late pregnancy, occurring usually during the last two months, which is marked by more or less severe intermittent convulsions, followed by coma, which sometimes deepens even to a terminal stage. Occasional cases are not accompanied by convulsions or coma.

"Pre-eclampsia" is described as a milder form of eclampsia, or as eclampsia in its initial stages.

The incidence of eclampsia is given as from five per cent to less than one per cent of all pregnancies, the occurrence being more frequent in colder climates or in the colder months of the year. The cause of the disorder is unknown.

This disease has serious effects upon many organs of the body; including the kidneys, liver, and brain, together with the lungs, heart and spleen. Maternal death may result from pulmonary edema, cardiac failure, or cerebral hemorrhage. The average mortality rate in severe eclampsia is given at about twenty per cent, with fetal mortality exceeding thirty per cent. If there is careful prenatal care and observation, the beginnings of pre-eclampsia and eclampsia can usually be controlled. In cases of severe eclampsia the following treatments are usually indicated by the authors:

1. Control of spasm by sedation, etc.
2. Attempted restoration of normal liver and renal function.
3. Termination of the pregnancy.

Moral Aspect: There is no moral difficulty in the usual case of real eclampsia, since this does not normally occur until very late in pregnancy, and the fetus is then viable and labor may be induced at the time and by the method of choice of a competent obstetrician.

However, if eclampsia does occur before the fetus is viable and does not readily respond to treatment, some obstetrical texts advise immediate termination of the pregnancy, even though there is no hope that the fetus can survive outside the uterus.

In the present state of the medical knowledge of eclampsia, such a procedure must be viewed as direct abortion and in violation of the uniquely divine prerogative of absolute dominion over human life. The procedure cannot be justified under the principle of double effect because, as the clinical facts are presented, the evil effect (the removal of the fetus from its vital environment) is necessarily directly willed, since it is envisioned as a necessary means to producing the good effect (the control of the eclampsia). As Adams and Cameron observe: "It is generally recognized that the most effective treatment for eclampsia is the termination of pregnancy."[147] Such an approach, however, before the fetus has reached viability, is simply direct abortion and thus unacceptable from a moral viewpoint.

This is the only moral evaluation that can be drawn from the present clinical knowledge of eclampsia. As research in placental function advances, new knowledge might possibly introduce some modification of the moral dimension. Ernest Page has pointed out that the placenta probably holds the key to most of the major unsolved problems in obstetrics. He notes that nearly every physiologic and biological change occurring in a pregnant woman is a result of placental activity, and that what is known about this vital organ "seems very little indeed when compared to our ignorance about placental physiology and biochemistry."[148]

Theologians have speculated on the possibility of operative interference in severe eclampsia before viability under the principle of double effect, basing their speculations on two questions: the accurate moral significance of the placenta in the maternal-fetal relationship, and the possibility that toxemia might be due to a malfunction of a pathological placenta.[149] On the medical side Berger and Cavanagh have done some speculative but highly controversial research at the University of Miami, suggesting the possibility of a pathologic myometrium-placental inter-reaction as the source of toxic elements[150] and Bartholomew, with his group at Emory, has done a great deal of work on this problem.[151] But these and other studies have not yet provided a sufficient medical basis for approaching the pre-viability eclamptic crisis under the principle of double effect, nor is there any positive indication at this time that a future solution might lie in that direction.

In those cases where eclampsia or pre-eclampsia occurs before the seventh month and is fatal to the fetus in utero, obviously, the dead fetus may be removed at the discretion of the obstetrician.

In cases presenting a history of this type of toxemia in successive pregnancies, with more or less danger to the mother and sometimes stillbirth for the fetus, sterilization has been suggested. Some have sought to defend this procedure under the principle of totality, proposing that in such circumstances the entire generative system has become pathological, even though each of its constituent parts is sound; and that the surgical removal or suppression of one of its parts would be done as a therapeutic procedure in a generative system which is diseased as a whole.

However, one cannot recognize eclampsia as a pathology of the generative system. It is rather an exacerbation of a vascular disease in the presence of pregnancy, and therefore a sterilization by invasion of the generative system, in these circumstances, could not be looked upon as other than a directly contraceptive sterilization, and therefore contrary to Catholic teaching.

Hyperemesis Gravidarum

Hyperemesis gravidarum is described as excessive or pernicious vomiting during pregnancy. It has been traditionally listed as one of the toxemias of pregnancy, although some have taken exception to this classification, since it seems to be actually a psychogenically exaggerated form of the usual "morning sickness" which occurs in about two-thirds of all pregnancies from about the middle of the second month until the end of the third month. Depending on the intensity of the psychogenic factor, it may persist as occasional vomiting throughout the entire pregnancy.

The acidosis, starvation, dehydration, etc., associated with vomiting can render the condition serious. In acute toxic cases death can occur within weeks. The fetus usually survives the illness, and if delivered is found to be normal and well-nourished.

A moral problem arises from the fact that some obstetrical authors still indicate termination of the pregnancy in hyperemesis gravidarum, even if the fetus is not viable, although this is less frequent in the more advanced obstetrical writings.

Moral Aspect: Since severe hyperemesis gravidarum usually occurs in the early months of pregnancy, it must be pointed out that the termination of the pregnancy before the fetus is viable is obviously immoral, as an act of absolute dominion in human life.

The principle of double effect cannot be employed here, because the evil effect is not merely permitted, but necessarily willed, because it is a real means to attaining the good effect. Such a procedure is again reducing fetal life to a mere means of preserving the maternal life.

This casual approach to the life of the fetus which was common enough in some quarters, reflected not only a shallowness of moral appreciation, but also poor obstetrical practice.

This is evident, for example, from the fact that The Margaret Hague Maternity Hospital reports on two hundred and ninety cases of hyperemesis gravidarum, over a ten-year period, with no maternal deaths and only one therapeutic abortion; while the Misericordia Hospital in Philadelphia reports only one maternal death from hyperemesis gravidarum over a period of twelve years, with no therapeutic abortions.

Note the following extremely significant comment of Cunningham, Professor of Obstetrics and Gynecology of the University College, Dublin, in his *Textbook of Obstetrics*:

Abortion was formerly much practiced, but with the treatment described above it should never be necessary. In neglected cases coming late for treatment, with the liver already badly damaged, abortion will not only fail to save life, but will actually hasten the end. A study of hospital records shows clearly that in those institutions where abortion is not practiced, deaths from true hyperemesis have virtually disappeared; whereas in institutions where abortion is done, the disease still carries a considerable mortality.[152]

Epilepsy

Epilepsy is generally recognized as being aggravated by pregnancy, but the *Journal of the American Medical Association* summarized an article by Dr. H. Dunsdale in the *British Medical Journal* reflecting the opinion that, with modern therapy, the epileptic woman should not be discouraged from pregnancy unless her attacks are difficult to control in the non-pregnant state;[153] and James McClure, of Ohio State University Medical Center, reviewing twenty-eight pregnancies in conjunction with grand-mal epilepsy, concluded: "As far as can be determined, idiopathic grand-mal epilepsy is without effect on pregnancy except for the patient with status epilepticus; the effects of pregnancy on idiopathic epilepsy are unpredictable. In this series the majority of patients had more frequent attacks with pregnancy."[154]

Not only is therapeutic abortion morally unacceptable under any circumstances; but while reserving judgment pending further studies, it is interesting to note that neither the usual antiepileptic drugs nor the maternal seizures seem to be harmful to the fetus.[155]

Erythroblastosis Fetalis

Erythroblastosis fetalis is a hemolytic disease of the newborn, usually manifested by anemia, jaundice, the presence of detectable antibody on the infant's red cells, and the presence of a large number of nucleated red cells in the circulating blood. The complication is normally not serious for the mother, but carries a high fetal mortality.

As early as 1923 Ottenberg postulated the theory that isoimmunization was in some way responsible for erythroblastosis fetalis, but it was not until 1940 that Landsteiner and Wiener published experimental data supporting the theory.

The Rh antigen was identified as present in the blood stream of a large majority of the human race, and it was discovered that the antigen of the red blood cells of an Rh positive fetus can probably cross the placental barrier at times, and bring about the production of antibodies in the blood stream of an Rh negative mother. These antibodies, produced either in the manner just described or by transfusion of Rh positive blood, having reached a sufficiently high titer, can recross the placenta and produce erythroblastosis fetalis in this or some subsequent pregnancy.

Without going into the genetic background of the Rh factor or the complexities of the lipoprotein chemical structure making up the varieties of the Rh antigen, we concern ourselves here only with the moral problems that can sometimes arise in connection with erythroblastosis fetalis.

Moral Aspects: As the physician studies the Rh background of his pregnant patient and carefully watches for any rise in her antibody titer curve, he will find the present literature on the subject opening the question of whether he should elect to do a therapeutic abortion, or induce labor after viability, or do exchange transfusion on the infant at delivery, and/or do a subsequent contraceptive sterilization on the mother.

The indications described for any one of these choices, or for a combination of them, vary greatly in the present medical literature, depending on the state of research on the subject or the school of thought which the individual writers adopt.

Therapeutic Abortion: We have already pointed out that there is no so-called "medical indication" which warrants the direct killing of an unborn baby.

Induced Labor and Exchange Transfusions: As the physician watches the progress of his patient, whether or not he wants to induce labor after viability and/or do exchange transfusion is entirely up to his sound professional judgment. From a moral viewpoint he need only keep in mind the maximum safety for both the mother and the child.

Exchange Transfusion in Utero: An optimistic dimension to the Rh problem has followed upon the diagnostic technique of successful amniocentesis and spectophotometry of the fluid to serve as an index of fetal hemal distress.[156] Pushing this invasion on into the fetal abdomen, William Liley first injected red cells with limited success[157] and subsequently Karlis Adamsons, Jr., exposed one leg of an unborn fetus through the mother's abdomen and transfused directly into the femoral artery, and subsequently experimented with the indwelling catheter approach.[158]

While investigation along these lines continues, it should be noted that success in these undertakings has been encouraging but limited. It is certainly true that when amniocentesis indicates that a particular fetus cannot survive until viability any procedure, no matter how risky, is advantageous and morally acceptable. In the early stages of development of these techniques, however, the Denver group sounded the following significant caution:

If the individual has not had a previous stillbirth, the pregnancy should be managed by conventional methods, i.e., premature delivery, because the technique of intrauterine transfusion is not sufficiently safe to weigh favorably against the risks of intrauterine death. Intrauterine fetal intraperitoneal transfusions should be regarded as being in the investigational stage, and other more adventurous undertakings for attempting intrauterine fetal transfusions should be confined to animal experimentations.[159]

Contraceptive Sterilization: Contraceptive sterilization is discussed at some length in other sections of this book. It is sufficient to say here that directly intended contraceptive sterilization is immoral, whether in the presence of Rh complications or in any other circumstances.

We might add here that the prediction of erythroblastosis fetalis would certainly supply sufficient reasons for a husband and wife to observe periodic continence according to the theory of ovulation rhythm.

In consideration of these moral aspects of erythroblastosis fetalis, the following words of Heffernan and Lynch are significant:

Many therapeutic abortions are done today for problems involving the Rh factor. This attitude is untenable. The grave danger of interrupting a pregnancy on the basis of rising titers or other assumed warnings of erythroblastosis developing in the infant is well brought out in a paper of Kendig and Waller published in 1948. The first patient had had an erythroblastic baby and in the pregnancy under consideration the titers were rising rapidly. One of the 'leading authorities' on the subject advised that interruption of the pregnancy seemed advisable. Pending this decision, the patient withdrew her permission for a therapeutic abortion and subsequently delivered a healthy infant who was Rh negative.

The second patient had had two spontaneous abortions and two severe erythroblastic babies and during the pregnancy in question had been advised twice to submit to a therapeutic abortion. Close to term she required a caesarean section and was sterilized. Her baby was a perfectly healthy Rh negative infant. Interruption of these pregnancies would have destroyed normal children.

The. Rh factor has produced its share of abnormal children. However, the positive constructive approach (not the destructive approach of therapeutic abortion) to the problem has salvaged a gratifying number by the exchange transfusion.[160]

Gaucher's Disease

A summary of the pertinent elements of the typical Gaucher's syndrome as found in the medical literature describes the disease as a rare metabolic error wherein the cells of the tissues which form the framework of the lymph glands, the red bone marrow, and the spleen become abnormally modified and multiplied. This immediately results in the enlargement of the spleen, liver, and lymph nodes and in modification of the bone marrow. Infiltration of other organs has likewise been observed.

There has been no satisfactory treatment for Gaucher's disease. Infants succumb rapidly, but when the onset is in adult life the condition is more likely to be chronic and slow-moving. Attendant anemia may cause weakness; and bone lesions may give rise to lameness, fractures, and skeletal pain.

Captain (MC) W. J. Hoja, of the Fitzsimmons Army Hospital, published a searching study of Gaucher's disease in pregnancy, including a review of the literature and two successful cases of his own. While the article refers to one theoretical and admittedly unlikely set of circumstances in which the author would approve therapeutic abortion (which would not be morally acceptable), his other conclusions are presumably clinically wise and certainly morally sound. He stated that:

> Therapeutic abortion is not indicated by Gaucher's disease or its complications. Pregnancy does not adversely affect Gaucher's disease and the disease does not adversely affect pregnancy. Splenectomy is effective in the treatment of certain complications of Gaucher's disease and may be performed during pregnancy if necessary.[161]

Hansen's Disease

Hansen's disease, or leprosy, is so rare in the United States that many American obstetric texts make no mention of it in connection with pregnancy, or at most give the condition only a passing reference. Until fairly recently, however, it was generally held that although the disease had no effect on pregnancy and children born of parents with Hansen's disease were not likely to contract it if reared in a healthy environment, the pregnant state was viewed to have very adverse effects on the course of the leprosy.[162] The result of these views has been that when pregnancy is identified in the presence of Hansen's disease, some clinicians advise destruction of the fetus in order to help the mother in spite of the fact that medical ideals, as well as moral rectitude, would dictate every effort to preserve the lives of both, or at least not to kill either one.

Moreover, King and Marks point out that with the advent of the sulfone group of drugs, the whole picture has changed remarkably. Although the evidence does not indicate that these drugs are totally effective, their efficacy in preventing aggravation of leprosy during pregnancy has been well illustrated by the Carville studies.[163]

Hepatitis

There seems to be general agreement among clinicians that pregnancy, at least in the third trimester, is a complicating element in hepatitis, whether of the virus A or virus B variety. It is likewise generally accepted, however, that in no case is therapeutic abortion the answer to this complication. The present literature might be summarized by saying that early pregnancy does not present a problem serious enough to warrant its termination and, in later pregnancy, termination is more dangerous than continuation of pregnancy. Long, Boyson and Priest observed that emptying the uterus does not solve the problem and while they stated that: "Hepatitis is an infectious disease dangerously complicating pregnancy," they added that: "Conservatism in the handling of the pregnancy is recommended."[164]

Adams and Combes of Southwestern report the former pessimistic views of many authors who felt that viral hepatitis in pregnancy increased maternal mortality and that therapeutic abortion should be done. They suspect, however, as a result of their carefully controlled study of thirty-four cases of this complication at the Parkland Memorial Hospital (Dallas) that such a pessimistic outlook is unscientific and probably based on an unintentional bias arising from retrospective analysis of the most severe cases; and they report: "Our results indicate that a favorable outcome may usually be anticipated for the woman who develops hepatitis during the course of pregnancy."[165]

Here, as in so many other instances, therapeutic abortion becomes less acceptable in the medical context as the science and art of medicine advance, even as it is never acceptable from the viewpoint of the Church.

Hodgkin's Disease

Hodgkin's disease, a pathology of the lymph nodes and also of non-nodal lymphatic tissue, is of unknown origin and is viewed as generally fatal. Whether it is an infectious granuloma or a true malignant neoplasm of the lymphatic tissue has been a matter of medical debate and not pertinent here. A therapeutic regimen of x-ray, nitrogen mustard, some of the newer chemotherapeutic agents and supportive care may induce remissions of the disease and certainly makes the patient more comfortable. In the presence of pregnancy, therapeutic abortion has often been done.

Aside from the fact that therapeutic abortion is morally unacceptable, it is interesting to note the following observations from the Sloan-Kettering Institute for Cancer Research and the Cornell Medical College:

> The influence of pregnancy on the Hodgkin's disease has been a source of controversy for many decades. The physician facing the problem in his practice can turn to the medical journals and find support for any view that his prejudices may lead him to favor, from the most favorable to the most dire. Early articles generally supported the view that pregnancy exerts a detrimental influence on Hodgkin's diseases producing an exacerbation of symptoms often with tragic consequences. However, as physicians encountered patients with Hodgkin's disease who tolerated pregnancy quite well, articles began to appear questioning this opinion.[166]

The following year Hennessy and Rottino reviewed thirty-five cases of Hodgkin's disease occurring over an eighteen-year period at St. Vincent's Hospital in New York with the following comment:

Opinions regarding the influence of pregnancy on Hodgkin's disease have led to diverse recommendations for treatment of pregnancy. One group of investigators advises its termination. One writer believes that in addition the patient should be sterilized. Nagel, who first followed this practice, later revised his opinion. Many, however, have recommended non-interference with pregnancy; our experience lends support to this view.[167]

Here, again, it must be emphasized that quotations such as these are not meant to turn a moral treatise into a clinical manual. They are merely offered as demonstrative of the fact that many procedures which are morally unacceptable, from the viewpoint of the Catholic Church, are likewise at least medically questionable.

Hydatidiform Mole

Hydatidiform mole is described as a grape-like conglomeration of vesicles arising as a lesion of placental tissue and consisting in a proliferation of the chorionic epithelium. It is a benign tumor or neoplasm which renders the placenta unsuitable as a nutritive agent. When the condition involves a large portion of the placenta the embryo, if it has ever developed, dies. It is more usual that in a pathologic examination no remnants of either a fetus or the amnion can be found but, as Titus points out, in other instances embryos and fetuses were seen in various stages of development and an exceptional pregnancy may go to full term with sufficient unaffected placental tissue to supply the fetal needs.[168]

In about fifty percent of the cases the uterus is remarkably larger than it would be at a given stage of normal pregnancy, but it is frequently smaller, or even of the size anticipated for a certain period of gestation. Because of the usual signs and symptoms the preoperative diagnosis is often incomplete, threatened, or missed abortion.

Treatment indicated in the literature includes dilatation and curettage for some stages of hydatidiform mole and abdominal hysterectomy and even hysterectomy with the mole in situ for other special cases.

Moral Aspects: The medical literature on hydatidiform mole suggests matter for moral comment in that two points are stressed: first, that the uterus should be emptied as soon as the diagnosis of hydatidiform mole is reached and secondly, that in the presence of a suspected mole it is frequently difficult to rule out the differential diagnosis of a living pregnancy. Rubin and Novak list the extent and rapidity of uterine expansion as indicative signs of hydatidiform mole, together with absence of fetal movement or heart sounds, albuminuria and edema in early pregnancy, bloody discharge, unusually large amount of gonadotropic hormone in the uterus and (confirming sign) the discharge of the characteristic grapelike vesicles.[169]

Titus advises manual evacuation by the vaginal route if cervical dilation is adequate; otherwise hysterotomy, but hysterectomy only under most extreme circumstances, and in the presence of incontrovertible evidence either of the coincidental occurrence of chorionepithelioma, or at least deep uterine wall extension or perforation by the tumor growth and immediate histopathologic examination of tissue for evidence of malignancy (cf. Titus, op. cit., p. 287).

Some have raised the question: "Is the mole a distinct human life?" Admittedly the identification of a new and distinct human life in embryonic form is not a simple problem. From the viewpoint of some fetal physiologists whose evaluative orientation begins with the blastoderm and looks forward, the mole itself, as a living organism arising from the union of ovum and sperm, might somehow be viewed as a distinct human conceptus, even though placental. To most obstetricians, however, and to the theologian whose evaluative orientation looks toward the immanent activity and teleology of the organism, the mole itself, as a neoplastic type of placental accretion, is rather something which arose from a once living but now presumably perished embryo; and hence the mole is not viewed as a new and distinct, howsoever deformed, human being. Hence, considerations such as those concerning baptism or abortion do not relate to the hydatidiform mole itself.

If hydatidiform mole which has advanced to such a state that it is incompatible with the presence of a living fetus is diagnosed, dilation and curettage, hysterotomy or even hysterectomy are morally acceptable and indicated, according to the medical indications.

If, however, the uterus even probably contains a living fetus, expectant treatment must be maintained until a positive diagnosis of hydatidiform mole is established and the presence of a living fetus is ruled out.

The situation becomes more delicate in those relatively rare cases in which hydatidiform mole is suspected to be present together with a surviving twin pregnancy. In such a case surgical interference would have to await the viability of the surviving fetus as long as the maternal life was not in imminent danger from the presence of the mole. If the maternal danger became imminent one could, under the principle of double effect, institute procedures for the removal of the mole, even though the surviving fetus would then perish. Although the usual obstetric text refers to this situation as being extremely rare, several cases of this type have been reported in the periodical literature.[170]

Idiopathic Thrombocytopenic Purpura

Any blood disorder which predisposes to hemorrhage is likely to be a dangerous complication of pregnancy and thrombocytopenic purpura, with its significant reduction of platelet count, prolonged bleeding time and poor clotting is a blood disorder which has been looked upon as a contraindication to pregnancy since the turn of the century.

Dr. Leon Tancer of Beth Israel Hospital (New York), however, after reviewing the literature and analyzing his own experience in these cases, submitted the following as a more modern obstetrical approach:

> Should a patient with a history of idiopathic thrombocytopenic purpura be advised to conceive? If she is pregnant, should the pregnancy be interrupted? The answers to both questions depend on the incidence of maternal complications and the maternal mortality rate. Premature separation of the placenta and maternal hemorrhage did not occur more often in the collected cases than would be expected in any un-

selected group of pregnancies. The maternal mortality of 5.5 per cent is no greater than could be expected from a group of non-pregnant patients with idiopathic thrombocytopenic purpura. Thus pregnancy may be advised in the patient with a history of idiopathic thrombocytopenic purpura, and pregnancy should not be interrupted because of idiopathic thrombocytopenic purpura.[171]

By way of a moral comment on these views of Dr. Tancer, it might be pointed out that, depending on all the circumstances of the individual case, the physician might want to advise that the patient seek to avoid future pregnancies by morally acceptable means; and that the total unacceptability of therapeutic abortion is based rather on the certainty of fetal mortality than on some danger to the maternal health, or the absence of such danger.

Kyphoscoliosis

Patients with kyphoscoliosis (hunchback), because of their pulmonary deficiencies and cardiac limitations, have often been viewed as subjects for therapeutic abortion and contraceptive sterilization. It would appear, however, that they can successfully bear children with proper obstetric care. Dugan and Black, of Western Reserve, concluded in this regard: "Women with kyphoscoliosis compare favorably with those not so afflicted in their ability to conceive, to deliver vaginally, and to withstand successfully postpartum complications."[172]

Leukemia

Types of leukemia, as a neoplastic proliferation of leukocytes particularly in the bone marrow, spleen and lymph nodes, are differentiated primarily according to the predominant type of abnormal cells. Acute leukemia may be fatal within six months while chronic cases may survive for some years. Some clinicians have viewed pregnancy as a factor sufficiently complicating to be avoided or terminated in chronic leukemia.

Not only would therapeutic abortion be contrary to the moral teachings of the Catholic Church, but Lee, Johnson and Hanlon, after an analysis of the pertinent case histories at the

Mayo Clinic, reported that: "In chronic leukemia we were unable to find any convincing evidence that the course of the disease is influenced in any way by pregnancy, except that early gestation imposes an obstacle to vigorous treatment," and they conclude that: "the obstetric care should be based on the principles applicable to any pregnancy. Since definite evidence is lacking that pregnancy has a deleterious effect on leukemia, and since the stress of interrupting a pregnancy may be greater than that of parturition, we believe that interruption of pregnancy is not indicated."[173]

Likewise Mulla, in reporting a case and having reviewed the literature on acute leukemia and pregnancy, concluded that:

It is evident from the foregoing case and those reviewed that pregnancy does not essentially alter the course of acute leukemia, fatal uterine hemorrhage being rare. Although leukemia is a definite cause of premature birth to the offspring, a leukemic mother has never been known to give birth to a leukemic child. Interruption of the pregnancy is of no benefit and may hasten the death of the mother.[174]

Lupus Erythematosus

Systemic lupus erythematosus is primarily a disease of the connective tissue which merits consideration here because its occurrence is so predominant in women of child-bearing age. Clinical investigation of the disease has increased in recent years because prolongation of the lives of these patients, due to treatment with the adrenal corticosteroids, has allowed for more extensive observation. Although the generic notion of lupus has been thought of mainly as a dermatologic disorder, this form is referred to as "systemic" or "disseminatus" to emphasize the fact that there is likely to be extensive involvement of the viscera as well, due perhaps to an abnormal immune mechanism which results in the production of antibodies against the patient's own tissue.

There was scant reference to lupus erythematosus in the obstetric literature until Donaldson, of the University of Washington, reported on eight cases in 1952, indicating the mutual inter-reactions of pregnancy and the disease entity. In a follow-up study, twelve years later, involving 134 patients and including 191 pregnancies, Donaldson concluded that pregnancy exerted no effect on acute lupus erythematosus in half of the cases, that improvement occurred in a third of the cases and that the disease was aggravated in a sixth of the group.[175]

In view of the fact that abortion, although totally unacceptable in the Catholic concept of medical ethics, has been considered in some clinics to be a medically indicated therapeutic measure in lupus erythematosus, the following observation of Donaldson and deAlverez is significant:

> Therapeutic abortions were carried out for acute SLE in twelve instances. It is important to note that only one patient's condition was improved following therapeutic interruption of pregnancy. In the remaining eleven patients the disease process was either unchanged or was reactivated postabortally. Of great significance is the fact that three of the twelve patients whose pregnancies were interrupted, died.

This fact, together with their other observations, led Donaldson and deAlverez to the conclusion that: "termination of pregnancy really has no place in ameliorating the disease process."

Similarly the group at the Mayo Clinic, after a study of the patients there between 1954 and 1960, concluded that: "From this study it appears that pregnancy does not pose a substantial threat to the subject with systemic lupus."[176] Indeed, Friedman and Rutherford, of Columbia, have gone even further to say, in regard to their own studies, that: "The question of therapeutic abortion has been touched upon, and although insufficient data are herein available, it is implied that no real beneficial effect on the course of the disease may be accrued thereby. In fact, the exacerbation which may likely occur post-operatively in already seriously ill patients may indeed be the proverbial last straw."[177]

Multiple Sclerosis

Although multiple sclerosis is a clinical entity which remains somewhat shrouded in mystery, the symptoms of sensory disturbances, transient weakness or loss of muscular control, with spontaneous remissions but progressive worsening, all indicate the presence of multiple lesions of the brain and spinal cord. The presence of pregnancy has been viewed as deleterious in multiple sclerosis and therapeutic abortion is often recommended. This destructive approach to fetal life is not only morally unacceptable, but one gets the impression from the literature that it may not even be medically advantageous to the mother.

Sweeney reported on his series of twenty-two cases in 1953, which had risen to fifty-one cases by 1958, and it is his impression that no definite effect on the course of the disease could be attributed to pregnancy;[178] and similar conclusions based on larger series have been reached by Tillman in the United States, Millar and McAlpine with their group in England, and Muller on the Scandinavian Peninsula, as collected and reported by Garvin at the University of Chicago. Garvin concluded that:

> With the present evidence available it is not medically justified to recommend against pregnancy on the grounds that pregnancy will increase the chance of an exacerbation, or that it will alter the course of the disease, or that there will be adverse effect on the child. Therapeutic abortions are not indicated in patients with multiple sclerosis based on the small number that have been reported.[179]

Myasthenia Gravis

Myasthenia gravis, as a chronic neuro-muscular disorder resulting in weakness and low fatigue threshold of the voluntary skeletal muscles (aggravated by exercise and partially alleviated by rest), has been identified as a clinical entity for almost 300 years. The medical literature of the eighteenth and nineteenth centuries contains many reports of therapeutic abortion, particularly in the first trimester, in the presence of myasthenia gravis. But with the advent of the anticholinesterase drugs in the 1930's and the subsequent control of symptoms, the trend has been away from abortion.

This change has been reflected in the standard obstetric texts as well as in the current literature.

Plauché, of the University of Mississippi, reviewed the British and American literature on the subject of myasthenia gravis and pregnancy from 1938 to 1946. Although his implication that therapeutic abortion might be justified in some rare cases is morally unacceptable, the following quote from his summary is significant: "The patient with myasthenia gravis may be advised that, although hazards exist, she can frequently maintain adequate control of the disease through pregnancy and confinement and produce a healthy infant."[180]

Chronic Polyarthritis

Pregnancy in the presence of chronic polyarthritis is sometimes viewed as a medical indication for abortion, particularly in Denmark, on the supposition that abortion will actually be beneficial toward relieving the arthritis. This practice is not only morally disordered, but a study by Felbo and Snorrason (*Ugesk Laeger*, July 7, 1960) demonstrated that the assumption on which it is based is likewise medically unsound.[181]

Psychiatric Illness

In recent years there has been an increasing tendency on the part of some physicians to view therapeutic abortion as an acceptable part of psychiatric therapy. In 1951 Overstreet and Trout observed the beginnings of this tendency, noting that: "There has been a decrease in the number (of therapeutic abortions) done in toxemias of pregnancy, heart disease, tuberculosis and other medical diseases, but an increase in the number done for psychiatric reasons."[182]

In 1953 Dr. George Fulty, in his Chairman's Address to the Section on Neurology and Psychiatry of the Southern Medical Association, likewise noted this rising tendency and speculated as to whether some of it was due to the psychiatrist's too strong identity with the patient, fearing any trauma in the patient's somewhat delicate psychic balance. As Dr. Fulty expressed it: "[The psychiatrist] may even go so far as to recommend a termination of pregnancy, based on his own emotional feelings rather than on sound judgment."[183] Harden Brauch and Reiser were among the many who feared that, in any given case of psychiatric illness, an abortion may precipitate greater illness instead of alleviating the situation at all. They pointed out that:

". . . the stress of interrupting the pregnancy, with the physical incapacity, the difficulties stemming from the legal safeguards surrounding the operation, and the severe guilt reactions that often are an indication of the ambivalence of the mother toward pregnancy—these might be as contributory to a psychotic episode as the delivery itself would have been."[184] Arbuse and Schedtman had expressed the same doubtful misgivings. They had written, in 1950: "There does not seem to be any one condition which absolutely indicates interruption of pregnancy . . . Abortion, per se, is unquestionably a shock. It may be conceivably more detrimental than continuation of pregnancy."[185]

Obviously this brief sampling of the literature is not presented as a complete review of current psychiatric opinion, and other quotations favoring therapeutic abortion would not be hard to find. Rosenberg and Silver, of the Palo Alto Medical Research Foundation, pointed out that those psychiatrists who are known to recommend abortion frequently do receive more consultations than their more conservative colleagues. Their report likewise tends to prove, very strongly, that abortion has no place of value in psychiatric therapy.[186]

From a moral viewpoint it is evident that no psychiatric complication on the part of a mother could ever constitute justification for a physician to kill her unborn child. And a cross-section of the current medical literature merely confirms that, in the eyes of many psychiatrists, here is one more situation in which good moral theology is likewise good medical practice.

Phocomelia

Phocomelia is described as a fetal malformation consistent with normal mental development but characterized by a dramatic and deforming foreshortening of the arms and, in some cases, the legs; with the hands and feet likewise deformed and attached almost directly to the trunk of the body. The condition was relatively rare until the thalidomide catastrophe of the late 1950's and early 1960's. It was at this time that thalidomide, a pharmacological sedative, was synthesized in Germany and marketed in Western Europe and the United States to a limited degree. When suddenly thousands of babies were being born with phocomelia, the causal agent was identified as thalidomide taken in early pregnancy.

The drug was withdrawn from the market, but the damage had been done. Sensationalized in the popular press, the facts became focused in the public emotions in 1962 when an American mother who had taken thalidomide sought to have a legal abortion. Refused in the United States, she flew to Sweden, amid great publicity, to have the abortion. A similar case was likewise sensationalized in the press when a Belgian court acquitted a mother who, a week after her phocomelic daughter had been born, poisoned the infant with barbiturates.

The moral disorder involved here should be evident. Indeed the immorality of infanticide is the same whether it is done by way of therapeutic abortion after rubella or other compromising infections, or because of undesirable hereditary problems (such as in Huntington's chorea), or by post-natal poisoning of the infant (as in the Belgian case). The killing of an infant after delivery instead of before delivery may have different legal implications and emotional overtones, but the immorality of the act is the same in either circumstance.

Polyarteritis Nodosa

Polyarteritis is a collagen disorder with lesions of the arterioles and medium sized arteries of almost any area of the body and is sometimes looked upon in some clinics as a medical indication for therapeutic abortion. This is not only morally unacceptable, but likewise seems to be medically questionable. Although little is known about the disorder, Arthur Haskins, answering a question submitted to the *Journal of the American Medical Association*, wrote that: "There is no evidence that a general worsening of this or other collagen disorders is caused by pregnancy . . . In general, polyarteritis nodosa should be treated in pregnancy as in the nongravid state. Therapeutic abortion is not indicated."[187]

A similar opinion comes from Felba and Snorrason of Denmark. Writing in *Ugesk Laeger* (July 7, 1960) they submit their findings regarding the induction of therapeutic abortion in the presence of polyarteritis, which they report to be a fairly common practice in Denmark. After their experience of fifty cases they conclude that this so-called medical indication for therapeutic abortion is scientifically unsound.[188]

Pulmonary Tuberculosis

From about 1850 until 1925 many physicians looked upon pulmonary tuberculosis as a medical indication for therapeutic abortion. This, of course, was never acceptable in the Catholic concept of medical ethics; and although between 1925 and 1950 this destructive approach to fetal life came to be viewed as medically outmoded, it is evident from the literature that too many physicians still held to the outdated concepts of an earlier generation in this regard. Rosenbach and Gangemi, of the Henry Phipps Institute at the University of Pennsylvania, lamented this fact in 1956 when they wrote:

> Too often one hears chest physicians, well trained in tuberculosis treatment, recommend therapeutic abortion during the first trimester of pregnancy in active cases or advise in inactive cases a two to five year waiting period before pregnancy. The figures in this series indicate that neither of the recommendations is based on facts. Certainly, pregnancy would not be recommended in the active case, but, should it occur, therapeutic abortion is not indicated. Moreover, with proper medical treatment and obstetric care, there should be no deleterious effect from the pregnancy on the tuberculosis process.[189]

At exactly the same time as Rosenbach and Gangemi published their report, Sidney Jacobs wrote, in the journal: *Diseases of the Chest:* "The Aphorism of Young: 'If a virgin, no marriage; if married, no children; if pregnant, no delivery'—was formulated at a time when it was generally believed that pregnancy could not be tolerated by the tuberculous woman. So pessimistic an attitude is not justified."[190] Reviewing the antibiotics and other available therapeutic measures at the middle of the present century, Jacobs concluded that: "The patient may be truthfully reassured that with adequate therapy, she will continue to improve despite the pregnancy, may be delivered of a normal child by the same maneuvers that would be used if she did not have tuberculosis, and will be non infectious by the time of confinement."

This tone grows constantly stronger in the literature. A comment by Myers, in 1963, serves as a summary: "There is no well documented evidence that tuberculosis has a deleterious effect on pregnancy or vice versa . . . If the pulmonary tuberculosis is brought well under control there is no contraindication to a reasonable number of subsequent pregnancies."[191]

Renal Disease and Hypertension

Renal disease, nephritis, or Bright's disease include a number of pathologic states, acute or chronic, accompanied by protein, casts, or sometimes blood in the urine; arising from inflammatory or degenerative lesions of the kidneys with concomitant disturbances of the vascular system.

There is no doubt that the combination of some forms of renal disease and pregnancy is likely to pose a formidable clinical crisis, and for this reason those physicians who do not hesitate to destroy fetal life in the interest of maternal safety frequently adopt therapeutic abortion as the most accessible avenue of escape from the problem. The situation is far more challenging, demanding and difficult for those physicians whose reverence for human life—the life of the mother and the life of the child—precludes the direct destruction of either life.

Yet in 1948 Brugsch and Brodie of Tufts Medical College wrote that: "During the course of the last twenty years the attitude of the medical profession toward the interruption of pregnancies in kidney disease has changed from frank pessimism to one of guarded optimism."[192]

Cunningham, writing of chronic kidney disease complicated by pregnancy, observed that: "Dangerous symptoms, in patients under treatment, seldom appear before the 30th week, and even at this early stage there is some hope of survival of the fetus."[193] And Heffernan and Lynch wrote that: "patients with chronic nephritis and hypertension complicating pregnancy may be conservatively treated today with proper diet, rest, and the use of hormone therapy, thoraco-lumbar sympathectomy and the administration of vascular anti-spasmodics, far more safely than by the interruption of pregnancy with its possible attendant hemorrhage and infection."[194]

Tenney and Dandrow maintain that hypertension alone is "a rather benign complication of parturition" and is not responsible for any severe trouble for either the mother or the baby. They allow, however, that this, complicated by renal disease, is a very serious medical complication frequently terminating in spontaneous premature labor, and would advise against these patients becoming pregnant when kidney damage is extensive.[195]

A distinguished team of specialists at Harvard reported a dramatic case of a woman with chronic renal disease who had developed severe azotemia in the last trimester of pregnancy, as follows: "With consideration of the known deleterious effects of maternal uremia on fetal survival, hemodialysis was attempted in the hope of improving fetal environment and obtaining a live infant at thirty-six weeks of gestation. There appeared to be little additional risk to the mother in delaying delivery for an additional three weeks under close medical observation . . . Having been maintained with intermittent hemodialysis for three weeks, she was delivered of a viable infant."[196] This kind of obstetrical patience and courage, looking always only to the safety of both mother and child, is the pride of the medical profession and the fulcrum of its advance against disease and death.

Maternal Rubella

Rubella, or German measles, is described as an acute exanthematous disease, accompanied by fever and rash, and caused by a virus. The incubation period is from one to three weeks, followed by mild fever, sore throat, etc., together with an eruption of red papules disappearing within a week.

The effects which maternal rubella may have on a fetus, particularly if contracted during the first trimester of pregnancy, have been highlighted by observations made during the 1941

Australian epidemic of German measles.

In such cases the fetus is liable to manifest certain malformations at term, such as cataracts, deaf-mutism, microcephaly, heart lesions, dental defects, or glomerular scelerosis.

As a result of these and other observations, many obstetrical writers advise therapeutic abortion for the mother who contracts rubella during the first three months of her pregnancy. Note the following as an example:

> *Eastman:* However, it is my own feeling that if the attack of rubella has been observed by a dependable physician and the validity of the diagnosis is beyond question, and provided that the disease occurred in the first three months of pregnancy, therapeutic abortion is justifiable if the mother and her husband do not want to assume the obvious risks involved.[197]

Looking through the literature to try to establish the incidence of fetal malformations following rubella, one can almost exhaust the entire range of percentages. This would lead one to conclude that the incidence is simply not known. Hussey made the following notable observation in this regard:

> *Hussey:* Entirely apart from religious or philosophical considerations, therapeutic abortion seems unjustified for scientific reasons. The truth of the matter is that there is still too much uncertainty regarding the risks induced by rubella in a pregnant woman. Thus, in their thorough review of writings on the subject, Krugman and Ward find that the disease entails a risk to the baby (abortion, stillbirth, or malformation) of something between ten per cent and ninety per cent. With a spread that large in the estimates, scientific evaluation of the place of therapeutic abortion had better wait for further studies.[198]

And further studies dramatically confirmed Hussey's 1954 warnings. The October 12, 1957 issue of the *Journal of the American Medical Association* carried an editorial pointing out that the common belief among many pregnant women "and even some physicians" regarding the inevitability of congenital malformities was based on fallacy.[199]

In the same issue of the same journal, Greenberg, Pellitteri and Barton report on their more carefully controlled observations of rubella in pregnancy. They point out the fallacies of earlier studies and conclude that the earlier recommendations of therapeutic abortion are not medically justified.[200]

And all of this received further confirmation as a result of the analysis of the 1958 Dallas-Fort Worth epidemic. Regarding this epidemic, Kantor and Strother of Baylor wrote that: "these experiences reveal that if the pregnancy did carry to term, induction of an abortion would have destroyed eighty-five normal children in order to prevent eleven being born with deficiencies."[201]

Moral Aspects: While it is unnecessary to repeat that the practice of so-called "therapeutic" abortion, as direct abortion, is in violation of moral law, one cannot refrain from raising the question as to how such a procedure, which is both a moral and a medical monstrosity, could achieve a fairly wide acceptance in the medical profession.

In the first place the accepted meaning of "therapeutic abortion," even in the medical profession, is the termination of fetal life in the interests of the maternal health. Abortion in cases of rubella, as Father Gerald Kelly, S.J., pointed out, is more accurately described as "fetal euthanasia."

Kelly's comment still applies to similar situations.

From the moral point of view there is no such thing as an 'indication for therapeutic abortion.' This is true in general, because 'therapeutic abortion' means direct abortion, and direct abortion is a direct taking of innocent life—and this, apart from divine authorization, is murder. As for rubella in particular, it is just as fully murder to kill an unborn baby lest it be born defective as to kill a defective child already born of a defective adult. In fact, if we could distinguish degrees in these various types of murder, we might say that therapeutic abortion for maternal rubella is worse than the killing of defective children and adults because in this case the unborn baby is by no means certain to be defective.[202]

The fact that the research efforts of the 1960's have almost eliminated the rubella problem through the discovery of effective vaccines does not make these moral and ethical observations obsolete. As the rubella problem decreased, the use of diagnostic amniocentesis for the prenatal diagnosis of fetal abnormalities, with its attendant risks and intended abortions, has filled the rubella void. The same ethical considerations and moral evaluations apply.

Varicose Veins

Dilation and tortuosity of the superficial veins of the legs may be due to defective venous valves or as compensation for some deeper circulatory obstruction such as thrombophlebitis. The varicosities, however, which are likely to occur during fifteen to twenty per cent of pregnancies may also be found in the vulva and vagina and are quite different in their pattern and pathogenesis and are thought to be aggravated by the increase of hormones during pregnancy as well as by mechanical factors.[203] The problem increases as the pregnancy progresses, and usually regresses after delivery, but is likely to be more severe with succeeding pregnancies.

Robert Nabatoff, of the Prenatal Varicose Vein Clinic of Mt. Sinai Hospital (New York), has published extensively in this field and his findings indicate that the condition need not give rise to any serious moral problems. He points out that the use of elastic supports is effective and:

> Since any untoward operative reaction may involve the fetus as well as the mother, our policy has been conservative. The use of hormones has not proved necessary. In an occasional instance of an unusually troublesome varix, injections of sclerosing solution may be given, but these have rarely been necessary.[204]

Even though the complication may become more severe after many pregnancies, neither contraceptive sterilization nor therapeutic abortion would be acceptable from the Catholic viewpoint; although periodic continence might be suggested. Nabatoff adds, in this regard:

> An occasional patient who has had many gestations will develop huge varices. This individual should be discouraged

from having further pregnancies . . . Therapeutic abortion has not been necessary thus far in our clinic, because even the largest varices and their complications have proved amenable to effective control during pregnancy.

The Hemorrhage of Pregnancy

Obstetric hemorrhage is one of the most common causes of both medical crises and moral problems in pregnancy. Several of the problems which are dealt with in the following pages can be classified according to abnormal location or behavior of the placenta (threatened and inevitable abortion, abruptio placentae, placent praevia) and according to the ectopic site of implantation (tubal, secondary abdominal, ovarian and cervical pregnancy).

In general the moral approach to these problems is the same as the medical approach: toward conservative and expectant treatment when possible, transfusion, bed rest, and whatever the medical armamentarium offers to achieve both maternal safety and fetal salvage.

In the presence of hemorrhage, however, the moral distinction between direct and indirect abortion is of paramount importance. To directly kill the fetus, or to uproot it from its site of implantation, is never morally acceptable. There will be cases, however, where indicated measures to control hemorrhage do endanger the fetus, and cases in which the very area of maternal tissue which is the site of implantation is likewise the site of dangerous hemorrhage and will have to be excised irregardless of the conceptus. In such circumstances the principle of double effect provides the background for a moral judgment regarding what course to pursue.

Abruptio Placentae

Abruptio placentae can be described as the premature separation, in part or wholly, from the uterine wall, of the placenta implanted at its normal site. The condition results in hemorrhage at the site of detachment, and may be called "invisible" or "concealed" hemorrhage because confined within the limits of the placenta; or may be "external" or "revealed" hemorrhage, when the swelling tide of blood lifts the placental membrane off the uterine wall at some point, and thus escapes through the cervix and into the vagina.

Hypertension or trauma in the presence of degenerative changes in the blood vessels due to toxemias or certain other diseases can trigger the mechanism of abruptio placentae. The degree of separation may vary from being slight and harmless to complete separation; with maternal mortality nearing thirty per cent. Severe hemorrhage is listed as occurring about once in eight hundred pregnancies, sometimes between the twenty-eighth week and delivery.

According to the site, nature, and extent of the hemorrhage, everything from watchful waiting, rupture of fetal membranes with premature delivery, to caesarean section and hysterectomy, is advised.

Moral Aspects: When, as is more usual, abruptio placentae occurs near term or at the onset of labor, when the fetus is viable, the obstetrician will do all that he can to save the lives of both the mother and the child. It is obviously permissible, in the hope of controlling the hemorrhage, prematurely to remove a viable fetus from the uterus in whatever way sound medical judgment indicates.

If, however, abruptio occurs before the fetus is viable, the following points are of great importance:

1. When the maternal hemorrhage is mild and not endangering the mother's life no steps can be taken which would even indirectly expose the life of the fetus to any considerable danger. The element of proportion in the principle of double effect is to be carefully considered here. One of the conditions which must be verified for the correct application of the principle is that there be a due proportion between good that is intended and the evil that is permitted. To avert a slight danger from the mother by a procedure which would expose the fetus to considerable danger would violate this proportion.

2. Even if the hemorrhage becomes serious, the directly intended removal of a non-viable fetus from the uterus

is direct abortion and is never permitted.

3. When the maternal life is in danger from hemorrhage it is morally permissible to try to control the bleeding by drug therapy or tamponade, even if it is foreseen that this will result in premature labor or in fetal death from some other cause. The principle of double effect is employed here. The good effect, directly willed, is the control of the hemorrhage by morally licit means. The evil effect, fetal death, is not directly willed, although it is foreseen as at least a probable, if not certain, side effect of the attempt to control the hemorrhage.

4. Laparotomy and amputation of the uterus in the presence of a fulminating placento-uterine hemorrhage, even with a non-viable fetus in situ, is permitted under the principle of double effect. The good effect, directly willed, is the control of the hemorrhage by means of the removal of bleeding tissue. The evil effect, the death of the fetus, is foreseen but merely permitted.

5. The removal of a dead fetus at any stage of development is obviously not wrong. Moreover, in the case of complete separation of the placenta, the fetus is already dead or will be dead within a few minutes after complete placental detachment. It is important to note that under such circumstances immediate steps may be taken to remove the fetus, if this is indicated, even though some trace of fetal life remains. Such a procedure puts the fetus in no worse an environment, and is therefore permitted.

Another important consideration in this connection is that immediate delivery after complete placental separation, while not involving direct abortion (never allowable for any reason), does offer a notably better chance for baptism of the fetus.

Placenta Praevia

Placenta praevia is described as the implantation of the placenta on the lower segment of the uterine wall, within the zone of dilation, sometimes wholly or partially covering the os uteri. The condition is said to occur approximately in one out of every hundred and forty pregnancies. Maternal mortality is estimated between five and eighteen per cent, with fetal mortality running about fifty per cent.

The hemorrhage usually does not occur before the eighth month. By then the lower uterine segment has considerably developed and there is a constant upward pull on its fibers. Thus the area occupied by the placenta implanted here is enlarged and under strain, and the placental growth is not proportionately increased: hence the hemorrhage. The prognosis is always serious.

Moral Aspects: Since a placenta praevia does not usually enter upon a stormy course until after the fetus is viable, the moral complications are greatly reduced. After viability the uterus may be emptied at the discretion of the obstetrician, and in the manner most advantageous to both the mother and the child.

However, sometimes hemorrhage comes on before viability, and in this case some of the standard obstetrical texts indicate direct abortion. This is, of course, not consonant with the right order or the norm of morality. Note the following quotations from obstetrical texts:

> As a rule the uterus should be emptied by the most conservative method as soon as placenta praevia is diagnosed. There are rare exceptions, e.g., when a couple is very desirous of having a baby and are willing to assume the risk.[205]

> Treatment during Pregnancy before Viability . . . If a central or partial placenta praevia is found the uterus must be emptied.[206]

> Plans should be made for termination of pregnancy as soon as a diagnosis of placenta praevia has been definitely established. These need not be carried out in those cases where hemorrhages have been slight and infrequent, the period of viability of the fetus is near, and the placental attachment is scant 'partial.'[207]

By way of comment on these quotations it is sufficient to reiterate the simple principle: that all so-called therapeutic measures which directly attack the life of the fetus are immoral.

Moreover, it should be noted that in placenta praevia, as

in many other complications of pregnancy, moral as well as obstetrical difficulties are not infrequently precipitated by what might be called a "trigger happy" attitude, or the desire to rush in and institute drastic measures when a conservative period of treatment and watchful waiting would obviate many of the difficulties, both moral and obstetrical. Note the following observations of Marchetti:

> The mortality resulting from obstetric hemorrhage is for the most part preventable . . . There is no hurry to confirm the diagnosis of a suspected placenta praevia once the patient is in the hospital. At any time during pregnancy, only profuse and continuous bleeding demands immediate and correct diagnosis and treatment. Overstreet and Traut have shown that in ninety-five per cent of women admitted to the hospital for antepartum bleeding in the last trimester of pregnancy, the bleeding will subside spontaneously within the first twenty-four hours of observation if one refrains from any early manipulation.[208]

Threatened, Imminent and Inevitable Abortion

Obstetric texts identify the various stages of spontaneous abortion as threatened, imminent and inevitable. Since definitions of these stages may vary somewhat in the accepted medical dictionaries and obstetrical texts, we have selected the most common understanding of each term for moral comment on the indicated procedures associated with these stages of obstetrical difficulties.

Threatened Abortion: Threatened abortion is described as the appearance of signs of the premature expulsion of the nonviable fetus. This stage is identified by the beginning of minor blood loss and minimal pain. The normal procedures prescribed include bed rest and pharmacological attempts to control and remedy the situation and save the pregnancy. Obviously there is no moral problem in such obstetric directions.

One might ask, however, to what lengths must a mother go in terms of bed rest, expense and general inactivity to try to preserve a pregnancy in the presence of threatened abortion. The moralist's answer to this question is based on the principles of charity, reinforced by the mother-child relationship. The infant is in extreme physical danger and therefore the mother is obliged to undergo very serious hardship as long as there is real hope of saving the infant.

Inevitable Abortion: Inevitable abortion is described as a condition in which a combination of untoward factors has so affected the fetal attachments and environment that the expulsion of the non-viable fetus has progressed to such a point that the abortion cannot be prevented. The usual sign is rupture of membranes in the presence of a dilated cervix, accompanied by bleeding and pain.

Litzenberg neatly summarizes the suggested standard treatment as follows:

"When abortion becomes inevitable, time, effort, blood and health of the patient will be conserved by terminating the pregnancy promptly . . ."[209]

Moral Aspects: Since in the presence of incipient inevitable abortion the fetus may not be dead or completely separated from its site of nidation, the artificial hastening of its inevitable expulsion presents some moral difficulty. As the case is described, the fate of the fetus is sealed prior to this intervention by the obstetrician, and yet there may be the possibility that the artificial acceleration of the process may hasten fetal death.

Perhaps because the moral evaluation of this question so much involves trained obstetrical judgment being brought to bear on each individual case, the moral theologians have not written extensively on the precise and delicate point at issue here.

All theologians would agree that once there has been total separation of the placenta from the uterine wall with concomitant fetal death, the fetus may be removed in any obstetrically indicated way. On the other hand, regarding the case wherein the placenta is the site of some relatively minor hemorrhage, theologians and obstetricians are in complete agreement on the need for conservative treatment.

Inevitable abortion, however, is different from either of these situations, wherein there is moral and obstetrical unanimity regarding proper procedure in the presence of an evidently detached placenta, on the one hand, and an evidently attached, but slightly hemorrhaging placenta, on the other hand. But the transition is not instantaneous. A placenta might be in the process of progressive separation for some time, and it is here that the moral problem arises.

We believe that during this progressing separation a point may be reached wherein the obstetrician rightfully judges that inevitable and advancing separation has so irrevocably progressed that to empty the uterus, in an attempt to save the maternal life, would not be actually destructive of a non-viable fetus, even in the event that some fetal life might still possibly be present. The hastening of fetal death is neither sought nor intended nor, in these circumstances, is it likely to be materially influenced by the acceleration procedure.

And yet a strong word of caution is in order. In the presence of even extensive uterine hemorrhage, the obstetrician will often feel incapable of judging that the separation is far advanced and inevitable. In such circumstances, interference by emptying the uterus would be totally unjustified.

Imminent Abortion: Imminent abortion is described as impending abortion in which bleeding is profuse, the cervix is softened and dilated, and the cramps are approaching the character of labor pains.

Eastman's comment on this crisis was as follows:

> Since an imminent abortion is almost certain to terminate in actual abortion, it is wise to hospitalize the patient at once. If bleeding and pain persist unabated for six hours, it is probably best to face the reality of abortion and encourage occurrence by injecting 0.5 cc. of pituitrin every half-hour, for six doses . . . If the patient is afebrile and the pituitrin does not succeed in making the pregnancy abort, the patient should be taken to the operating room and a curettage done, under anesthesia . . . If the patient is febrile, further temporization is obligatory, unless the bleeding is too severe to permit it. Whenever possible, the expectant treatment should be pursued in febrile cases until the patient has been afebrile for seventy-two hours.[210]

Moral Aspect: The above comment from Eastman might

seem, at first glance, to reflect an attitude too ready to terminate a pregnancy. It must be borne in mind, however, that it is impossible to exactly identify the moment at which a threatened abortion becomes an inevitable abortion.

Greenhill's comment is pertinent:

> We agree with Paine, Hertig, and also Rutherford that in most cases spontaneous abortion occurs as a result of a pathologic condition of the ovum incompatible with continuing pregnancy and that the clinical picture of abortion in such cases represents in reality a terminal phase of an already interrupted pregnancy.[211]

The moral evaluations of procedures in threatened abortion and in inevitable abortion have already been outlined. We believe that imminent abortion represents a transitional stage between these two, and that whether it should be treated, in an individual case, as threatened abortion or as inevitable abortion must be left to the immediate judgment of the conscientious and competent obstetrician.

In this connection attention should be called to the Shirodkar procedure, in which the incompetent cervix (dilated and membranes frequently protruding) is surgically closed with fetal salvage as a frequent result.

Pitocin and Ergot: Some moral comment is indicated regarding the use of pitocin or other ergotrate preparations in imminent or inevitable abortion. This pharmacological approach to serious maternal uterine hemorrhage is sometimes used in an emergency to control the bleeding by inducing contraction of the uterine musculature. A moral problem arises because these contractions not only tend to control the bleeding of the uterus, but will also likely sheer off the already separating placenta, thus hastening fetal death.

This clearly presents a case of double effect. The purpose of the medication and resultant contraction of the uterine wall is to control a dangerous hemorrhage. The consequent placental separation is an effect which is in no way intended as a means to achieving the good effect. Moreover, the therapy sometimes controls the hemorrhage without the contractions unduly disturbing the placenta.

The proper proportion between the good effect and the evil effect is inherent in the obstetrical crisis, for it is only in a true crisis that the therapy could be justified. Many obstetricians have pointed out that the ordinary treatment for hemorrhage is transfusion.

Ectopic Pregnancy

Ectopic pregnancy is described as any gestation developing outside of the uterus. Although the vast majority of such pregnancies are found in the fallopian tubes, there is also the possibility of implantation on the ovary itself, or in the abdominal cavity, or in the cervix.

Tubal Pregnancy: The various accepted classifications of tubal pregnancy, determined by the part of the tube in which nidation occurs (ampullar, isthmic, interstitial) are of no particular importance in the moral consideration of tubal gestation.

The important fact is that the implantation of an ovum in any part of the fallopian tube presents a serious pathological situation almost at once, due to the fact that the normal process of nidation of a fertilized ovum is advancing in a place which is neither anatomically nor histologically suited for this invasion.

Unlike the uterus, the tube is not equipped to form true decidua, and so the ovum immediately erodes the tubal musculature; and the invading villi can completely perforate the tube, or so weaken its walls that the danger of rupture rapidly becomes imminent. The invading villi are opening the maternal blood vessels, the enlarging gestation is straining against the lines of least resistance, and very soon one of several sequences may occur. The following are sufficient for our consideration.

Tubal Abortion: Most commonly the pregnancy ruptures into the lumen of the tube (usually between the sixth and twelfth weeks) and then is carried out through the fimbriated distal end of the tube and deposited in the peritoneal cavity.

Tubal Rupture: The invading villi may perforate the tube wall, or the weakened wall may yield to the growing pressure from within, usually triggered by the sudden opening of a large blood vessel or the clogging of the venous channels by the villi.

Moral Aspects: By the time that tubal pregnancy has advanced to a stage where it can be diagnosed, even if the diagnosis is only incidental to laparotomy for some other reason, the tube will usually have been so damaged as to constitute a serious threat to the maternal life. In cases where this usual eventuality is judged to be verified, the tube may be removed as traumatized pathological tissue. The principle of double effect applies. The theologian cannot make the general statement that whenever a tubal pregnancy is discovered the tube may be excised immediately. The pathology of the tube and the degree of danger attendant upon expectant treatment in each individual case is a matter for the obstetrician. There have been a number of cases of advanced tubal pregnancy reported in the medical literature. Between 1914 and 1959 there are ten cases wherein both mother and baby survived and seven of the infants were full-term.[212]

If one encounters a rare case of tubal pregnancy which has advanced to a stage approaching viability, it is obvious that the element of proportion in the principle of double effect has to be given very special consideration. In such a case special attention must be paid to the proportion between the risk of expectant treatment for the mother and the chances of soon delivering a viable fetus. Unless the danger to the mother notably outweighs the chance for fetal survival, expectant treatment would be the procedure of moral choice.

Secondary Abdominal Pregnancy: Tubal rupture normally occurs at the point of placental attachment, disturbing the maternal-fetal connections to such an extent that the fecundated ovum dies. However, if the maternal connections are maintained after rupture, it is possible for the baby to continue to develop between the layers of the broad ligament or in the peritoneal cavity. In these cases a large thin placenta may become attached to the proximate internal organs, drawing all or part of its blood supply from the viscera.

Moral Aspects: A secondary abdominal pregnancy must be permitted to advance, if possible, to viability. To directly remove it before viability is a direct killing of the fetus. However, under the principle of double effect, in the actual crisis of dangerous hemorrhage (which might occur at the placental site before viability) surgical intervention to control the bleeding is obviously permissible, provided no direct attack is made on the fetus.

Ovarian Pregnancy: Ovarian pregnancy is a rare form of ectopic gestation which can result if the implantation of a fertilized ovum occurs within the ovary. Only about a hundred authentic cases of ovarian pregnancy have been reported in the literature, and although early rupture is the usual termination, it is to be noted that a considerable percentage of ovarian pregnancies have gone to term.

Moral Aspects: If an intact ovarian pregnancy is diagnosed on the occasion of laparotomy, the moral picture resembles that of secondary abdominal rather than tubal pregnancy. Since, as has been pointed out, a considerable percentage of ovarian pregnancies have gone to term, it seems that the ovary can accommodate itself more readily than the tube to an ectopic gestation. Therefore, as long as rupture has not occurred and as long as the mother's life is not in imminent danger from her own traumatized tissue, one could not justify surgical intervention on the ovary while there remains some real hope of delivering a viable fetus in the future.

Cervical Pregnancy: Even rarer than an ovarian pregnancy, a cervical pregnancy results from the implantation of a fertilized ovum in the cervix. Studdiford believed that cervical pregnancy results from the inability of the fertilized ovum to reach the maturity required for implantation until it has dropped through the uterine cavity and reached the cervical canal.[213]

DeLee-Greenhill point out that many of these gestations are unrecognized because of early spontaneous abortion, that they rarely continue beyond the twelfth week, and that, should they continue, surgical intervention because of hemorrhage, rupture of the amniotic sac, or perforation of the cervical wall is usually necessary before the fifth month.[214]

The danger attendant upon the condition is the sudden profuse hemorrhage from the rupture of the thinned out cervix. In profuse bleeding, packing of the cervix and even total hysterectomy may be required.

From a moral viewpoint, a cervical pregnancy presents very much the same picture as a tubal pregnancy. Studdiford's emphasis on "the urgent necessity for early diagnosis in order to apply vigorous measures to avert the potential disaster attendant upon cervical pregnancy" supplies a background for a moral comment.

The immorality of a direct attack on the ectopic fetus, by simply removing it as a source of future trouble, is evident. But the possibility of surgical intervention upon dangerously pathological tissue, under the principle of double effect, also presents itself. The real source of danger lies in the fact that placental elements are invading the cervical tissue, and that some major blood vessels lie in the path of this invasion. Certainly a point is reached at which, in the judgment of a prudent obstetrician, the cervix is so traumatized by this invasion as to be dangerously pathologic tissue whose removal is now indicated irrespective of any future fetal development. At this juncture the principle of double effect certainly applies, and hysterectomy may be done.

A Note on Surgical Procedure in Tubal Pregnancy: Some of the moralists have stressed that, in cases of tubal pregnancy where surgery is indicated, the non-viable fetus must be left in situ, in the tube, until after the tube has been removed. These writers seem to imply that any removal of the fetus prior to removal of the tube is direct abortion.

Good and Kelly: Let us make it plain that one cannot, even for the desire to baptize the fetus, open the tube and remove the fetus, and then remove the tube. The tube must be removed with the ectopic pregnancy still in the body of the tube, and then the tube may be opened and baptism given.[215]

Bouscaren: It is one thing to remove the tube containing the fetus; it is another thing to remove the fetus directly. This distinction will be made clearer in the argument; but in the meantime it is necessary to emphasize the fact that only the first method of operating—namely, the removal of the tube itself, without interfering directly with the fetus—is the only method which is in any way defended in this thesis.[216]

Obviously, as Father Bouscaren points out in the context of the quotation just cited (and this is the case which he seems to have in mind), one cannot legitimately shell out the fetus and leave the tube, or even shell out the fetus with the hope of possibly being able to repair the tube. This would clearly be an abortive procedure. As the legitimate distinctions of moral theology continue to be obscured in the current context of utilitarian ethics, this particular procedure is being advocated in the interest of preserving the tube. However, it must be remembered that the entire radical procedure in tubal pregnancy, to be morally justified, must be based on the presumption that the tube itself is so pathologically affected here and now that surgical intervention on the tube itself is indicated. Moreover, to distinguish between removing a non-viable fetus from the uterus and from the fallopian tube is patently (from a theological viewpoint) to make a distinction without a difference. If, however, a skilled surgeon should recognize the probability of success in attempting to transplant a tubal pregnancy into the uterine cavity, without seriously adding to the mother's danger and at the same time securing some real hope for fetal survival, this would certainly be morally acceptable. At present such a procedure does not seem to be looked upon with any great optimism by obstetricians. It has, however, been successfully undertaken on at least one occasion,[217] and how far such a technique may be developed in the future is an interesting speculation.

Finally, a brief study of the histological structure of the fallopian tube indicates the real possibility of a section of the tubal wall being so traumatized in early ectopic pregnancy as to warrant the removal of that section, leaving the tube in situ after repair. In a case where these conditions would be really verified we see no moral difficulty in such a procedure. The principle of double effect would be applied in the removal of dangerously pathological tissue surrounding the site of fetal implantation.

This is a newer, and morally very delicate approach, to tubal pregnancy. If we are to be consistent with our moral principles regarding the inviolability of human life, then even here one cannot aim at the destruction or removal of the embryo as the purpose of the surgery, but the nature and purpose of the surgical technique must still be the removal of dangerously pathological maternal tissue.

Moreover, even from a gynecological viewpoint, the advisability of this approach has been much debated, as predisposing to further tubal pregnancies.

In matters involving such delicate, and not yet fully developed, operative techniques the theologian can only indicate the principles under which the morality of the procedures must be evaluated.

Induced Labor

Induced labor is understood as the initiation of the birth process by artificial or mechanical means at some period after the fetus is judged to be viable (i.e., capable of extrauterine life) and before the natural onset of labor at term.

This definition of induced labor is adopted and expressed here in order to facilitate the discussion of its moral aspects. Artificial induction of labor before viability is recognized as direct abortion.

Medical Indications for Inducing Labor: Obstetric writers list various organic and systematic diseases of the mother, particularly of a nephritic nature, as well as certain contingencies related to the pregnancy itself (such as abruptio placentae) as medical indications for inducing labor. The purpose of this is to ameliorate the maternal strain or complication, thus insuring greater safety for the mother, or for both mother and child.

The methods of inducing labor have varied from a purging dose of castor oil, through administration of pituitary extract, to rupture of the membranes. The respective merits of the various methods, used alone or in combination, do not concern us here. The choice of method will depend on the various elements present in each individual case.

Moral Aspects: The moral problem of induced labor arises out of the fact that premature delivery constitutes some danger to the fetus, more or less depending upon the period of gestation after viability at which labor is induced.

Eastman described a premature infant as:

> One which has been born so early in the course of gestation that its organs have not yet reached full development so that its chances of survival, although not entirely hopeless as in abortion, are less good than those of an infant which has enjoyed the full period of intra-uterine growth.[218]

DeLee and Greenhill point out that, for the child, the general mortality rate is from thirty to sixty per cent, depending upon the period of pregnancy and the indications which demand the intervention.[219]

The moral solution to problems of induced labor is to be sought in the principle of double effect. The good effect is the alleviation of the mother's condition and the lessening of danger to her, and often to the child also. The evil effect is found in the more or less serious danger to the life of the child.

In accord with the principle, granted that the fetus has reached viability, the two questions to be asked in each case are: first, is there any less dangerous method by which the good effect can be sought with reasonable hope of success; and secondly, is there a proportion between the danger warded off by the induction of labor and the fetal danger incurred by this procedure?

If the answer to the first question is in the negative and the answer to the second question is in the affirmative, there is no moral objection to inducing labor at whatever time after viability is most desirable in the judgment of a competent obstetrician.

Non-medical Indications for Inducing Labor: Cases of induced labor close to term for reasons of convenience or expediency unrelated to the clinical aspects of the case have not been unheard of. These vary from the depressing report of a doctor inducing labor in order to be able to begin his vacation on time to the more understandable desire of a husband, about to embark on a long military mission, to see his child before leaving the country.

Moral Aspects: An interesting observation on how this problem can change with advancing prenatal techniques is to be found in the following assay of the question in the *Journal of the American Medical Association* over twenty years ago. To the question: whether the increasingly common practice to induce labor for no other indication than the convenience of the attendant, or of the parturient, can be considered good obstetrical practice, the *Journal* replied, in part:

The answer is unquestionably that it is not good practice in general. One must, however, consider in this problem the following factors. 1. The group at Evanston Hospital, Evanston, Ill., found that it was perfectly safe to induce labor by rupture of the membranes if the patient was near term, the cervix was soft and effaced, and there were no contraindications such as malposition. 2. There is an increasing number of patients with very short labors with their first pregnancy and there are many multiparas who barely get to the hospital in time for delivery. 3. With the advantage of the sulfanamides, the antibiotics and better prenatal and intranatal care, there is now such a low morbidity and mortality that many procedures are probably done now that never would have been dreamed of twenty years ago. . .

Perhaps in a few more years we will consider this normal practice and until then accept an attitude of tongue-in-cheek toward it, rather than one of lifted eyebrows. Certainly the burden of proof of its safety is on the shoulders of those who practice early induction.[20]

Granted the proper maturity of the fetus and the presence of the proper physiological indications in the mother's anteparturient condition, such as would give assurance that the procedure would be perfectly safe for both mother and baby, induction of labor for non-medical reasons could be morally justified.

The principle of double effect is not invoked here because under the conditions described above there is no evil effect.

Although one should be alert to the danger of abuse in this procedure, one should likewise bear in mind that such cases of induction of labor may well contribute considerably to obstetrical progress, eventually increasing the margin of safety in the labor and delivery techniques. Thus we should hesitate to arbitrarily condemn the practice where safety is assured, even if the reasons for inducing labor are somewhat tenuous.

This philosophy was well expressed by Dr. Edward Bishop, from the Women's Division of the Pennsylvania Hospital, in the following words:

> The mere acknowledgment that complications can occur has prompted many critics to conclude that, since the practice of elective induction of labor is not wise for the tyro, it should not be contemplated by the experienced, or even discussed favorably by the teacher. Is it better, then, to reduce the practice of obstetrics to mediocrity by avoidance of any procedure that is considered new or improved, or is it better to accept a procedure which can be shown to be of value and to train ourselves to do it safely and well?[221]

To induce labor without the assurance of fetal safety, however, is permitted only for medical indications, or for some other reason vitally concerned with the safety of the mother or of the child.

General Surgery During Pregnancy

Occasionally, during the course of a pregnancy, some indication for general surgery to correct a condition unrelated to the pregnancy will arise.

The basic consideration in this situation first differentiates between elective and necessary surgery.

In general, elective surgery should be postponed until after the puerperium, on the supposition that the advantage of immediate surgery is negligible when viewed against the attendant danger to the developing fetus, as well as to the mother.

The immediacy of necessary surgery, on the other hand, is to be judged in the light of the principle of double effect. The good effect will be the surgical correction of some disease of the mother, thus extracting her from a more or less gravely dangerous situation. The evil effect will range anywhere from fetal death, as in the case of the surgical correction of cancer of the cervix during early pregnancy, to considerable or slight danger of fetal death or premature labor.

The element of proportion is of paramount importance here. One must estimate, weigh, and balance the dangers and advantages to both the mother and the fetus between expectant treatment for a longer or shorter time and immediate surgery.

Painless Childbirth

The pain of a woman in labor is proverbial in both profane and sacred literature, and modern obstetrics has made great advances in its attempts to alleviate and even eradicate these sufferings.

The modern pharmacologic attempts to reduce or eliminate the pains of childbirth go back to the historic use of ether and chloroform in the mid-nineteenth century, when James Y. Simpson was knighted for his use of chloroform to ease the labor pains of Queen Victoria. Since that time a great number of pharmacological approaches to the pains of labor and childbirth have enjoyed greater or less popularity. The process was long in a state of transition and today's procedures attempt combinations of the best elements of previous practices.

For the sake of clarity in presenting some moral evaluation of these advances, let us accept the term *painless childbirth* to mean the overall approach to the alleviation of parturient pain. Within this concept we distinguish *natural childbirth* as that approach to the problem of obstetric pain which relies mainly on the natural resources of the mother, with minimal help from chemotherapeutic measures, from *obstetric analgesia and anesthesia*, or the primarily chemotherapeutic or pharmacologic control of the pains of labor and delivery.

Natural Childbirth: The two most notable approaches to natural childbirth were found in the theories of the well-known British obstetrician, Grantly Dick-Read and the Russian School of conditioned reflex, based on the studies of Pavlov.

Read's theory may be summed up in the hypothesis that fear

is the chief pain-producing agent in otherwise normal labor, and a tense woman means a tense parturient passage. As Eastman pointed out, commenting on Read's theory: "Although the neuromuscular mechanism by which fear exerts a deleterious effect on uterine motility is obscure, the general validity of Read's contention is in keeping with common clinical experience."[222]

The Russian school followed Pavlov's theory that the cerebral cortex conditions the final form of pain perception, while the environment, through its influence on the cortex, modifies cortical function, and that thus women are conditioned to pain by the tradition that teaches them to expect pain as a necessary concomitant to childbirth.

Both schools seek to reduce or even eliminate the pains of childbirth by proper education of the pregnant mother, helping her to understand the physiology of childbirth and properly evaluate its emotional components. This approach is coupled with instructions and exercises in relaxation, muscle control and coordination, and breathing exercises adapted to the various phases of the birth process. The English group looks upon all these things as means to instill confidence and allay fear. The Russian school sees in them a means of prior conditioning of proper reflexes. Both theories seek, as a result, the more active participation of the parturient in the birth process with little or no pain. The proponents of neither theory claim total success and all would stand ready to supplement the process by some pharmacological analgesia. Conversely, the usual obstetric service, wherein the approach to control of parturient pain is primarily pharmacological, nearly always incorporates many elements of *natural childbirth* into its regimen. In modern obstetrics chemoprophylaxis and psychoprophylaxis are not mutually exclusive. The difference is one of emphasis. Today, in the United States, a combination of most of these elements has been popularized in the current Lamaze method, after Andre Lamaze.

Moral Comment: The specific concept of *natural childbirth* presents no moral problem at all. As Pius XII pointed out in a public address to a group of obstetricians and gynecologists:

"In itself it (natural childbirth) contains nothing that can be criticized from the moral point of view."[223]

It is true that some religious fundamentalists have envisioned a clash between science and sacred scripture in comparing the principles of painless childbirth with the first chapter of Genesis, precisely in the divine communication to the first mother of men: "In pain shall you bring forth children."[224] But as Pius XII pointed out: ". . . in punishing Eve, God did not wish to forbid and did not forbid mothers to make use of means which render childbirth easier and less painful . . . These words remain true in the sense intended and expressed by the Creator, namely, motherhood will give the mother much to endure."

The pharmacologic approach to relief of pain in labor and during delivery merits some moral consideration. Systemic anesthetics and analgesics can be expected to cross the placenta in some degree and are liable to affect the sensitive respiratory center of the fetus. Moreover, relatively slight degrees of maternal anoxia can be a danger to the fetus.

Earlier methods varied from a few inhalations of ether or chloroform, through combinations of nitrous oxide and oxygen, together with the barbituric acid derivatives (sodium amytal, pentobarbital, etc.) or reasonable doses of morphine and scopolamine or paraldehyde. These elements were used orally, intravenously, by inhalation or by rectum, and caudal anesthesia consists of injection of an analgesic agent into the caudal canal. Other regional and local nerve block techniques have been developed. Today more refined drugs are used intravenously, intramuscularly, or by inhalation. Caudal anesthesia, epidurals and regional nerve blocks are probably the most widely used techniques at this time, together with small doses of demerol, scopolamine, and the like.

Moral Aspects: The moral problem of obstetric analgesia and anesthesia is less vexing in those cases where, because of some obstetric difficulty or abnormality, the use of sedation is necessary for a safe delivery of the child. Here there is little difficulty in a correct application of the principle of double effect, with attention focused on the due proportion of risk to the mother and the infant with or without the use of particular analgesic and/or anesthetic procedures.

The moral problem is more difficult in the normal labor. Here the baby will usually be born satisfactorily without any kind of sedative medication, although the mother may suffer considerable pain.

This immediately poses the question for the moral theologian as to whether or not any anesthetic risk in obstetrics,, unless absolutely necessary, is an unjustified risk. In the following quotations from classic obstetric authors it is interesting to see their sound ethical evaluations ameliorate with the advances in medical technique:

> *Eastman*: Because of the difficulties presented by the several circumstances enumerated, no completely safe and satisfactory method of pain relief in obstetrics has been developed. As a consequence, it is sometimes alleged that the hazards of pain relief in labor offset its advantages. This is untrue. Quite apart from humane objectives, a vast experience has shown that obstetric analgesia and anesthesia, when judiciously employed, may be beneficial rather than detrimental to both baby and mother, at least in the over-all picture. The reason is this: pain relief forestalls the insistent importunities of the parturient and her family for premature operative interference; prior to the present era premature and injudicious operative delivery, thus provoked, constituted the commonest cause of traumatic injury to both mother and infant. In the case of the mother such injuries were occasionally fatal; in the case of the baby they were frequently so. The relief of pain itself, while commendable, would not justify the employment of methods which themselves are not without danger, were it not for the fact that they permit more meticulous, more gentle, and frequently easier deliveries, resulting in healthier mothers and more living babies.[225]

> *Titus*: In conclusion, it may be reiterated that there is no valid excuse, at the present time, for failure on the part of an attending physician to make some attempt to alleviate the sufferings of women in labor.

> The administration of amnesics and analgesics, as has been described, is a comparatively simple matter, and should

be possible under almost any circumstances of hospital or home deliveries. They are not always entirely safe, but their danger lies chiefly in over-dosage or administration so late in labor that the infant is affected from one or the other of these two cases or by the addition of inhalation anesthesia.

. . . Even in average normal labors the ease of the patient's recovery seems to be contributed to materially by sparing her the physical shock of the pain of labor.[226]

Litzenberg: Modern obstetrics dictates that the laboring woman should have all the relief compatible with complete safety, by securing analgesia (relief); amnesia (forgetfulness); or anesthesia (abolition of pain), all of which also protect against shock, physical or mental.[227]

Moral Evaluation: It is evident that the general use of analgesia and anesthesia in child birth is not without some hazard, particularly to the child. It is likewise true that in individual normal cases, properly selected procedures in the hands of a competent obstetrician reduce the risk to a minimum, so that the concomitant advantages (directly to the mother and indirectly to the child) are in proportion to these minimal risks and remote dangers.

In deliveries complicated by prematurity, prolapse of the cord, etc., greater fetal susceptibility to anesthesia heightens the risk to the infant. These cases demand of the obstetrician even more careful consideration of safety factors.

This brief comment suffices for the moral aspects of painless childbirth. The details must be left in the hands of the conscientious obstetrician.

Gynecologic Procedures and Suspected Pregnancy

Sometimes medical indications for dilation and curettage or other surgical invasion of the female generative tract arise in the suspected presence of an early pregnancy. Under these circumstances the physician is obliged to use every available means, such as pregnancy tests and consultation, to arrive at a reasonable assurance that the procedure will not harm or abort a living fetus. Note the following from directive 24 of the *Ethical and Religious Directives for Catholic Health Facilities:*

"In all cases in which the presence of pregnancy would render some procedure illicit (e.g., curettage), the physician must make use of such pregnancy tests and consultation as may be needed in order to be reasonably certain that the patient is not pregnant."

CHAPTER SIX

MEDICO–CANONICAL–
MORAL ASPECTS OF MARRIAGE

The Second Vatican Council (1962-1965), in its Constitution on the Church in the Modern World, proclaimed again the essential meaning of marriage, offering guidance and support to those who would preserve the holiness of the married state and foster its dignity. The Council pointed out that marriage has been established by the Creator and is qualified by the divine law, and that its benefits and purposes come within the ambit of that law. Its essence and meaning is established by God, and revealed to man; and is not subject to the vagaries of evolving human customs and social mores. Conjugal life, in both its pro-creational and relational dimensions, is protected in its integral meaning by the law of God, and this indeed for the realization of its own deepest fulfillment.

Some writers in the medico-conjugal field have viewed marriage as merely an evolving convention constantly changing throughout the history of mankind. Considering the modifications and distortions of marriage that have sometimes prevailed in various human cultures, one can more readily understand how these writers would come to this view. It is, however, aberrant from revealed truth and is more easily seen as such when one sorts out the accidental distortions from the fundamental concepts basic to that pattern of procreation and conjugal love which befits man in his highest aspirations and ideals. Moreover the Council obviously did not pretend to deny the facts of anthropological studies and the history of human culture, but only to proclaim that marriage finds its true meaning in the light of divine revelation.

This chapter is not meant to be a general treatise on marriage, but a commentary on those aspects of it wherein the physician (and consequently his patients) will be helped by a certain clarity of thought regarding certain pertinent moral and canonical concepts. Hence the emphases tend to become somewhat legalistic, morally analytical, and even biological. Marriage is much more than this, but even in these prosaic elements disorders may arise which, if not prevented or if left uncorrected, may satisfy certain short-range goals but ultimately destroy the happiness of marriage. Hence this chapter is designed to give the physician the technical moral and canonical knowledge to recognize these dangers in the lives of his patients, and to help his patients to avert them.

Canonical-Medical Aspects of Marriage

The physician will frequently be confronted with premarital and matrimonial situations wherein, if he is to evaluate the problem properly, he will have to possess a thorough understanding of some of the canonical aspects of marriage.

Definition of Marriage: Matrimony is defined as the lawful contract between a man and a woman, by which contract the exclusive and perpetual right is given and accepted, to those mutual bodily functions which are, of themselves, naturally suitable for the generation of offspring.

In order to arrive at a clearer understanding of the meaning of marriage it is helpful to examine, individually, each of the significant ideas in the definition:

Lawful contract: Marriage is a bilateral agreement between two people which is in accord with the natural, divine positive, and ecclesiastical law.

Some laws forbidding certain marriages are merely prohibiting laws, while others are invalidating laws. A marriage could be entered into contrary to some merely prohibiting law, and still be a real marriage, provided it was not also contrary to an invalidating law.

Civil laws invalidating marriage do not affect the marriages of the baptized, or even a marriage involving one baptized party, since such marriages come under the jurisdiction of the Church.

Invalidating civil laws do, however, affect marriages between non-baptized persons.

Exclusive and perpetual right: The right is perfectly bilateral, i.e., equal in the man and in the woman. It is an exclusive right, i.e., a union of one man and one woman. It is a perpetual right in the sense that the parties themselves cannot dissolve the bond.

To those mutual bodily functions, etc.: This means that the right is precisely and exactly the right to "perfect copula." "Perfect copula" is a technical term used to signify that act wherein the penis of the man, in a state of erection, penetrates into the vagina of the woman, and there deposits true semen. The meaning of "true semen" will be discussed subsequently.

The Canonical Concept of Impotence

Perfect copula, as defined above, is the actual matter of the matrimonial contract. If, for any reason, this act is impossible, impotence exists and there can be no marriage because there clearly can be no contract.

This is true irrespective of whether the parties are baptized or not. Among pagans marriage is a natural law or civil contract. Between the baptized, marriage is a sacrament, and it is the contract itself which is the sacrament of matrimony.

The question of impotence requires some detailed treatment because the physician will frequently be consulted with regard to whether or not impotence exists in a given case. Impotence is treated in the Code of Canon Law under Canon 1068.

Canon 1068: "1. Impotence, antecedent and perpetual, whether on the part of the man or the woman, whether known to the other party or not, whether absolute or relative, invalidates marriage by the law of nature itself.

"2. If the impediment of impotence is doubtful either in law or in fact, the marriage is not to be hindered.

"3. Sterility neither invalidates marriage nor renders it illicit."

Doubtful Impotence: In section 2 of canon 1068 the Church lays down the principle that the natural right to marry prevails over the doubtful impediment of impotence. Whether the doubt be a doubt of law: e.g., "Does the absence of the uterus constitute impotence?"; or a doubt of fact: e.g., "Is this man capable of perfect copula?", makes no difference. Unless the impotence is certain, the marriage is not to be hindered.

Obviously this principle allows for the possibility of invalid marriages. If impotence does, de facto, exist, the marriage is invalid. But to act on this principle is the nearest possible approach to right order.

Antecedent Impotence: Antecedent impotence means impotence existing antecedent to the marriage. To constitute the impediment the impotence must have existed before the marriage. A valid marriage is not dissolved by subsequent impotence.

Perpetual Impotence: Impotence is said to be perpetual when it cannot be corrected without serious danger to life or sanity, or without the commission of some crime.

Temporary impotence does not constitute an impediment to marriage, even if it exists at the time that the marriage is entered into. A girl with an impenetrable hymen can have her impotence corrected by minor surgery and therefore can validly marry even before the surgical correction of her impotence.

Note that if the impediment is to be considered present the impotence must be certainly perpetual and certainly antecedent to the marriage.

Absolute or Relative Impotence: Absolute impotence is a defect which makes the act of perfect copula impossible with all members of the opposite sex; e.g., the absence of the penis or the absence of the vagina. Relative impotence is a defect which makes the act of perfect copula impossible between two particular individuals, and so is an impediment to their marriage with each other only: e.g., disproportion of size.

Whether known or not: It is clear that whether one or both parties know of the defect or not makes no difference, since by impotence the essential matter of the marriage contract is absent, and hence there can be no contract.

Impotence and Sterility: Sterility is defined as the inability to generate children because of some physical defect; e.g., the absence of ovaries, even though one does have the ability to place the act of perfect copula. Sterility itself is not an impediment to marriage.

The Physiological Components of Impotence

As a background to a discussion of precisely what the physiological components of impotence are, the following considerations are of particular importance:

1. The impediment of impotence is derived from the natural law. Since the matter of the marriage contract is the right to marital intercourse, one who is incapable of true marital intercourse is, by that very fact, incapable of marriage.

2. The sacrament of matrimony is precisely the contract between two baptized and, as a sacrament, is completely under the authority of the Vicar of Christ and His Church, subject to the natural and the divine positive law. Moreover, since the contract is bilaterally indivisible, even when only one party is baptized the Church claims jurisdiction over the contract, but thus only indirectly over the non-baptized party.

3. The Church does not directly legislate the impediment of impotence but merely supplies an authentic declaration of the natural law.

4. The clearest authentice declaration regarding impotence is summarized in canon 1081, section 2; where the Code of Canon Law declares that matrimonial consent consists in giving and accepting: "the perpetual and exclusive right over the body, for acts which are of themselves suitable for the generation of offspring."

5. Thus the whole question of impotence is reduced to the meaning of the words: "acts which are of themselves suitable for the generation of offspring." The two sources for discovering the operative meaning of these words are the decisions handed down by the Holy See in particular marriage cases and the teaching of the canonists and moral theologians. These sources offer the following:

Minimum Physical Requirements for Potency as Regards the Woman: The minimum physical requirement for potency on the part of a woman is that she have a vagina that can be penetrated by the man whom she is to marry.

Absence of any or all of the post-vaginal generative organs—ovaries, fallopian tubes, uterus—does not constitute impotence, but only sterility. In the matter of perfect copula, the presence or absence of these organs does not affect the act itself. The same is true in the case of a woman who can admit peneration and semination in the vagina, but immediately ejects the semen.

A vagina that is so short or so narrow as to make penetration even of the corona of the penis impossible constitutes impotence unless the condition is remediable by surgery.

Anatomically the vagina is understood to extend from the vulva to the cervix; and although the impossibility of any penetration precludes the notion of a true marital act, in those cases where possible penetration is judged to be barely, if indeed actually, beyond the vulva, the physician must try to judge whether, in the given case, this can reasonably be called a natural marital act, i.e., a natural act which is, of itself, suitable for the generation of offspring.[228]

Vaginismus: Vaginismus is a sudden muscle spasm of the vagina with a siccative reaction of the vaginal vault which makes penetration difficult or impossible. It is of psychosomatic origin but is ordinarily not perpetual and hence does not constitute the impediment of impotence. Rubin and Novak point out that: "The prognosis of vaginismus is good. With proper treatment even the most obstinate cases of vaginismus can be cured within a period of a few days or at most weeks."[229]

Artificial Vagina: Construction of a vagina by plastic surgery, where no vagina or only a rudimentary one existed before, presents a question regarding canonical potency. Diverse aspects of the basic problem present themselves in the light of whether or not the artificial vagina connects with a functional or non-functional uterus, or ends in a *cul de sac;* and even in the latter case whether any internal generative organs are present or not.

Granted that the individual in question is fundamentally identifiable as a female, an artificial vagina constructed in its normal anatomical position is at least probably sufficient for potency. Therefore, according to the principle of canon 1068, the marriage of a woman possessing such a vagina is not to be impeded. She has, however, a grave obligation, at least in charity, to inform her intended spouse of her abnormality.

Whether or not such a vagina is joined to a uterus, or whether or not a uterus is present, does not substantially alter the canonical question as far as potency is concerned. Such considerations do not seem more pertinent in the case of an artificial vagina than in the case of a natural vagina. It is true that the Roman Rota decided impotence in a case involving an artificial vagina in 1929 (*Decisiones* XII, 1929, 406ff.). However, the constructed vagina was only about two inches in length. The Rota gave no general ruling, and the negative decision seems to have been based on the inadequacy of the plastic construction in this particular instance.

The opinion favoring potency is supported by three distinguished professors of Moral Theology: John C. Ford, S.J., of Weston College, Edwin F. Healy, S.J., of the Pontifical Gregorian University, and P. Tesson, S.J., of the Catholic Institute of Paris.

Father Tesson agrees with Professor Ombredanne, of the French Academy of Medicine, that the only requirement is that a vagina of reasonable dimensions be constructed in its proper anatomical area, allowing coitus with clitoridian contact and thus allowing for the allaying of concupiscence.[230]

Father Ford's conclusions in this matter are as follows:

> I do not know of any practical argument that can be brought forward to prove that a woman who has been successfully operated on is certainly impotent . . . before the marriage takes place. I do not know how anyone would set about getting an authoritative decision as to whether a woman in these circumstances is impotent, nor do I believe there is any obligation on anyone to attempt to get such a decision. In practice, however, many other considerations would determine the pastoral advice to be given on such a prospective marriage.[231]

Father Healy, agreeing with these opinions, adds explicitly the obligation in charity to notify the intended spouse of the abnormality. Moreover, in stressing the doubtful nature of the case, Father Healy makes reference to Canon 1031, no. 3, which directs a pastor to consult the local bishop before assisting at a marriage wherein some doubt exists as to the presence of an impediment.[232]

And since the pastor might feel justly disturbed if he were unable to fulfill this obligation, it would be proper for the physician to suggest that his Catholic patient, contemplating marriage, inform her pastor of the presence of the abnormality.

Minimum Physical Requirements for Potency as Regards the Male: The minimum physical requirement for potency on the part of the man is that he have a penis of such formation and capable of such erection that it can penetrate the vagina of the woman he is to marry, and there deposit true semen.

The absence of a penis, or one so distorted, either congenitally or traumatically, that it cannot penetrate the vagina and deposit semen, renders the man impotent.

Hypospadias: Hypospadias is the opening of the urethra on the underside of the penis. If this or any other anomalous position of the urethral opening is such as to preclude the possibility of ejaculating in the vagina, the impediment of impotence exists unless the condition is amenable to correction.

Aside from the possibility of surgical correction of hypospadias, Dr. F. Cone has observed that: "the simple expedient of using a condom with a hole in its top has been found to correct the faulty delivery in some cases of hypospadias."[233]

The main question here, of course, is whether or not a sufficient quantity of the ejaculate is thus deposited in the vagina to permit the act to be described as: "of itself suitable for the generation of offspring." Evidently such can sometimes be the case.

Regarding this matter, note the following comment of a late well-known professor of moral theology:

To me the use of a perforated condom appears as a facile

method of correcting a natural defect which would otherwise preclude marriage for a man stigmatized as impotent.
Any moralist would hesitate to forbid marriage to such an
individual capable of remedying hypospadias in so easy a
fashion.[234]

Paraplegia: Paraplegia is the paralysis of the legs and lower
trunk, affecting both motion and sensation. This condition frequently results in the inability to perform the act of copula. If,
due to paraplegia or any other cause, the man is permanently
incapable of erection and ejaculation, the impediment of impotence exists.

Priapism: Priapism is described as a persistent erection of
the penis, usually due to certain types of neurological disease or
trauma, unaccompanied by either venereal sensation or the ability
to ejaculate. Unless the condition is curable, as it is in some cases
by surgery (as, for example, when it is due to a tumor of the
spinal cord), the impediment of impotence exists.

Peyronie's Disease: Peyronie's disease is described as a fibro-
plastic induration of the penis, and is characterized by dense
fibrous tissue beneath the fascia which sometimes becomes calci-
fied, causing curvature during erection and making the act of
intercourse extremely painful. Various surgical and medical
measures have been tried in attempts to ameliorate the pathology,
but with limited success. Oral administration of para-animoben-
zoate has been reported as effective in many cases[235] and more
recently carefully controlled irradiation therapy, with testicle
shielding, has been done with considerable success.[236]

While the usual case of Peyronie's disease may make the act
of coitus extremely painful, it does not constitute physiologic
impotence. It might be noted here, however, that it would frequently constitute a sufficient reason for not rendering the marital *debitum*, particularly in view of the fact that its onset is
likely to be in middle age and hence subsequent to marriage.

Psychogenic Impotence: In cases where the individual is
venereally so sub-responsive that there can be no erection, or
it cannot be maintained until penetration or ejaculation; or in

cases which are so hyper-responsive that ejaculation always occurs before penetration, the disorder is usually not perpetual, and therefore need not constitute impotence.

The Meaning of "True Semen"

It has been pointed out that the authentic declaration of the Holy See regarding the essentials of the marriage contract contains the idea: "acts which are of themselves suitable for the generation of offspring."

In the conventional terminology of the canonists, the word, "true semen," as a technical term, is used to indicate the necessary components of an ejaculate in order that the act of intercourse be, of itself, suitable for the generation of offspring.

We have already seen that the absence of the post-vaginal generative organs of the woman does not render the marriage act, of itself, unsuitable for the generation of offspring. Notice that we are concerned here exactly and precisely with the act of marital intercourse itself, which is not the same as the actual generation of a child. Even though actual generation is precluded by post-vaginal physical defects, the act of intercourse itself is not altered.

The answer is not so clear cut in the question of the meaning of "true semen," or the necessary components of the male ejaculate. Here the precise difficulty comes down to this one point: whether or not the proper canonical concept of marital potency necessarily includes, in the ejaculate, something which has been elaborated in the testes.

In approaching this problem, it is of utmost importance to clarify the frame of reference. Almost subconsciously the physician may tend to look upon marriage as a purely clinical entity. Here it must be viewed as a natural law contract which is a sacrament between the baptized and within which the Church exercises her prerogative to teach and govern and sanctify the people of God. At the same time it is important to understand that the various and sometimes subtle dimensions of marital potency are not the subject of divine revelation, and that as these dimensions unfold with the advance of medical science, the Church seeks to weigh and sift and assimilate this new knowledge and theory, and to reconcile her ecclesial responsibility for the integrity of marriage with the advances in scientific thought of each succeeding age. Thus, in the canonical concept of impotence, there are some elements which are quite clear, and there are other areas where thought is still developing and far from definitive.

Eunuchism: The absolute minimum that is consistent with our present understanding of the marital act would seem to require some active testicular tissue in the male to fulfill the idea of marital potency. This is certainly the view of the Roman Rota (the Church's chief marriage tribunal) and thus we can say that the congenital absence, surgical or traumatic destruction, or total atrophy, of both testicles constitutes the canonical impediment of impotence.

The most authentic early declaration which touches upon this question is to be found in the *Cum Frequenter* of Pope Sixtus V, an official document sent to the Bishop of Navarre, dated June 12th, 1587, in answer to the question whether or not eunuchs should be allowed to marry.

The *Cum Frequenter* replied in the negative, and contained three reasons for this reply: that eunuchs are frigid by nature and unsuited for matrimony, that they are incapable of the marriage act, and that by their futile efforts to perform the marriage act and by their substitutions for it they themselves sin and cause scandal to others.

The interpretation of this document by the moralists and canonists was that in order to have "true semen," or in order to have "perfect copula" the ejaculate must contain testicular products. It is easy to see the logic of this conclusion, especially in view of the fact that the histology and endocrinology of the testes was not known for many years after the publication of the *Cum Frequenter.*

Moreover this interpretation continues to the present time, at least to the degree that it is commonly accepted that eunuchs, or those not possessing even one testis, are matrimonially impotent. Even when surgical castration has been done after puberty the castrate is, or soon will be, physically incapable of marital intercourse, since the endocrine function of the testes controls the activity of the accessory fluid-producing glands, such as the prostate, seminal vesicles, and Cowper's. This fact that in unusual cases a castrate may still be capable of erection and some ejaculation up to some years after castration, or that the effects of the testicular androgen can be substituted for by synthetic hormone therapy, does not alter the canonical aspects of the case. The castrate is canonically impotent.

The Question of Ineffective Seminiferous Tubules: It will be recalled that histologically the healthy testis is made up of seminiferous tubules, with the interstitial tissue interspersed, and that the epithelial cells of the tubules are in various stages of spermatogenesis, transforming progressively into spermatogonia, spermatocytes, spermatids, and spermatozoa; while the interstitial cells of Leydig are elaborating the internal hormone secretion which is directly picked up by the blood stream and is responsible for the secondary sex characteristics as well as sexual vigor.

A number of situations can occur wherein the seminiferous tubules do not produce spermatozoa, or anything else, such as in bilateral cryptorchism or after mumps orchitis; or wherein the products of the tubules are completely shut off from the ejaculate, as after double vasectomy or in the presence of complete nodular occlusion of both vasa diferentia. Meanwhile the interstitial cells of Leydig continue to secrete their hormonal products.

In such cases the man is capable of a grossly normal ejaculate, in which there is contained nothing that has been elaborated in the testicles.

Hence the question arises: is such an ejaculate to be considered as "true semen" and are such acts of intercourse able to be called "acts of themselves suitable for the generation of offspring"; or is such a man canonically potent or impotent?

Authorities for Impotence: The great weight of earlier canonical authority favored the view that impotence existed where the testicular component of the ejaculate was lacking. These authorities held that the man must have at least one testicle producing external secretion either from the testicle or the epididymis, even though the spermatozoa be dead or never fully developed, or completely lacking, or of insufficient number or vitality to fecundate an ovum; and that some of the testicular or epididymal secretion must be contained in his ejaculate.[237]

This was the more traditional opinion, and although it is a reasonable view and has been followed by the Holy See in some cases even in recent times,[238] it appears to depend too heavily on premises which were influenced by earlier and inaccurate medical theories. Indeed, prior to our detailed knowledge of the interstitial cells of the testicles, with their production and delivery of hormones directly into the system, the vasectomized male, deprived of sperm in the ejaculate, was thought by some to be comparable to the castrate in his ability to perform copula and in the quantity, viscosity, and general appearance of the ejaculate.[239]

Authorities against Impotence: There are authors of very great authority, both in the field of moral theology and in the field of canon law, who maintain that even if the vasa deferentia are bilaterally sectioned or completely occluded, the resulting absence of testicular secretion in the ejaculate probably does not constitute impotence.[240]

Moreover, aside from these classical authors, the trend of the more recent writers seems to be in this direction.

The argument of those who hold that the defect probably does not constitute impotence is normally based on the consideration that impotence, as an impediment to the external and social contract of marriage, should ordinarily be externally discernible, which is often not true in this case.

They point out, as we have seen, that neither side demands the presence of active sperm for potency and that the mere presence or absence of, let us say, spermatocytes, with their negligible amount of carrier fluid and without relation to the generation of a new life, cannot alone properly constitute an impediment to the marriage contract.

But since, as a matter of fact, a man lacking only testicular secretion in the ejaculate retains the power of erection and penetration of the vagina and is capable of an ejaculate that does not grossly differ from the normal, and since he is able to have marital intercourse which does foster mutual love and devotion and is effective in expressing and perfecting the relational aspects of conjugal life, it is difficult to see how, in the natural law, such a man can be said to be incapable of marriage.

Practical Solution: There is no doubt that each of the opinions outlined above is supported by sufficiently strong reasons to engender solid probability for it. Moreover, this is reinforced by the notable authorities supporting each opinion.

Meanwhile, when the physician is faced with this very practical problem, we would suggest the following procedures in cases where there has been double vasectomy or there exists complete bilateral nodular occlusion of the vasa deferentia, or sterility following mumps orchitis or some similar condition:

A. If at least one party to the proposed marriage is a Catholic, the physician might urge referral to the ecclesiastical authorities. This procedure is helpful for the proper external discipline of the Church, and for the future peace of mind and security of the contracting parties.

It is very likely that the judgment will be to the effect that the marriage is not to be impeded, because even if the lack of testicular semen in the ejaculate does constitute impotence there will nearly always be a doubt of fact: as to whether or not the condition is permanent. As a matter of fact the Holy See has expressly stated, in a private reply to a number of Bishops seeking guidance in this matter, that in the case of double vasectomy marriage was not to be hindered. (*Holy Office,* September 28, 1957).

Natural anastomosis of vasa which have been cut, partly removed, and with the ends buried in the tissue, has been reported and successful surgical anastomosis has been achieved in a number of cases. Mere ligation of nodular occlusion presents even less of a problem with regard to restoration of the lumen of the vasa.

B. If the proposed marriage is between non-Catholics, the physician himself must apply the norms of the natural law, as he knows them through the present development of canonical opinion and the practice of the Holy See. Since at present this admits of solid probability favoring marriage, the physician should not disturb the consciences of his non-Catholic patients in the matter, and should remain silent about the whole question until there has been a clearer and more authentic development of our knowledge of the natural law in this regard.

Hermaphrodism

An unusual combination of constitutional, hormonal, and probably hereditary factors during prenatal development can give rise to various types of bi-sexual and inter-sexual anatomical anomalies in the generative system.

This seems less strange if considered in the light of the sexually indifferent stage of embryonic development, when the urogenital sinus is common to the openings of the mullerian, wolffian, and metanephric ducts. It will be recalled that the solid epithelial outgrowths at the opening of the wolffian ducts give rise to the prostate in the male, and the rudimentary para-urethral ducts of Skene in the female. Moreover, Cowper's glands in the male and Bartholin's glands in the female both arise from evaginations of the urogenital sinus, and the genital tubercle becomes the male penis and the female clitoris. It is easy to see how any unusual influence along these lines of development could give rise to hermaphroditic anomalies.

Perfect Hermaphrodites: Perfect hermaphrodites are described as persons possessing all the generative organs, properly developed, of both male and female; so that the person can generate, or at least copulate, either as a male or as a female.

The existence of perfect hermaphrodites is usually denied, although some cases have been reported in the literature.

Canonical Aspect: It is at least probable that such persons cannot marry because it is probable that the natural law demands distinction of sex in marriage. Such a case, if discovered, should be referred to the ecclesiastical authorities regarding any question of marriage.

True Hermaphrodites and Gynandromorphs: True hermaphrodites are described as persons in whom there is an actual co-existence of male and female glands; neither fully developed but each present to such an extent that it is impossible to determine whether the person is male or female. Gynandromorphs are classified as a form of true hermaphrodites, and are described as persons whose gonads are composed of a mosaic of genetically male and female cells.

Canonical Aspect: True hermaphrodism is generally accompanied by complete sexual impotence. If this does not appear to be verified in an individual case, and the question of marriage arises, the case is to be referred to the ecclesiastical authorities.

Pseudohermaphrodites: Pseudohermaphrodites are described as persons in whom secondary male sex characteristics are superimposed on a genetic female, or vice versa. We would also classify as pseudohermaphrodites those who can be genetically determined as male or female, but who also possess some rudimentary or limited organs of the opposite sex, such as a man who has an ovary or a woman who has a testicle.

Canonical Aspect: In these cases of pseudohermaphrodism, by definition, the sex is certain, but there is usually some question of impotence. If impotence is certain, the individual cannot marry. If impotence is doubtful, the marriage cannot be impeded. These cases, however, should always be referred to the ecclesiastical authorities.

This brief and over-simplified classification is not presented as a comprehensive commentary on the vast number of variations in the problems of sex identification. Sex is accurately established by inspection of the external genitals in 99.9% of births, but in an estimated 1 in 1000 cases there is some question of sex identification.

Questions of equivocal sex identification may arise from intrinsic embryological defects, from abnormal endocrine activity associated with cryptorchidism in the male or ovarian androgenitalism in the female, and there may be various degrees and patterns of coexistence of ovarian and testicular tissue even in the presence of rather normal external genital morphology. The main areas of variability wherein equivocal indications of an individual's true sex may be found can be summarized as follows:

1. *External Genital Morphology:* The more or less clearly defined and identifiable external generative organs of one sex or the other.

2. *Internal Genital Morphology:* The presence of ovaries or testes, and of ovarian or testicular tissue, and other accessory structures.

3. *Chromosomal Sex:* At the turn of the century Murray Barr, of the University of Western Ontario, and his associates demonstrated a pattern of nuclear chromatin masses characteristically found in normal females. But later he himself and others pointed out that it is not safe to use the presence or absence of nuclear chromatin masses as a definitive indication of sex in ambiguous cases.[241]

4. *Gender Role:* Hampson and associates at Hopkins described the gender role of an individual as all the things which a person says or does to disclose himself or herself as a male or female. The gender role is built up through experience, casual learning, and explicit instruction. These investigators also point out that once the gender role is firmly established it is never entirely eradicated and that no even flagrant contradiction of body functioning and morphology may easily displace it.[242]

Moral Aspects: This almost schematic presentation of the elements of equivocal sex determination is presented only as an indication of the vastness and intricacy of the problem and as a background for the following moral considerations:

1. Everyone has a right to be a member of one sex or the other. The human race has received its pattern of sexual distinction ultimately from the Author of Nature. When anomalies occur which render accurate identification of sex problematical, the tendency has been to refer to the individuals in terms of "intersexuality" or "bisexuality"

and these notions find their way into the non-medical vocabulary as "half-man-half-woman" or "freak."

The moral implication here is that this type of thinking leaves the individual open to serious dangers of sexual abuses and morbid curiosities. Recent medical literature reflects a much truer and healthier approach to the problem by referring to it in terms of unfinished sexual development. This can be extremely helpful for both the individual in question, and for the family. The ultimate question of which sex is properly identifiable in a given case is a question for the medical specialist to answer, as best he can, in the light of present medical knowledge of the relative significance of the variables.

2. Everyone has a right to have the inconsistencies of his sexual anatomy corrected by plastic surgery and pharmacological therapy.

P. Tesson, S.J., as Professor of Moral Theology of the *Institut Catholigue de Paris* expressed the concept as follows: ". . . it is indisputable that a human being has always the right to fix himself or herself as clearly as possible in one of the two sexes of humanity. And the action of the surgeon who helps, by his art, those who wish to escape from the sexual indetermination imposed on them by nature, is perfectly justified."[243]

In cases where the sex variables are totally equivocal, the corrective approach may be toward either sex, depending upon the choice of the individual or, in the case of infants, the determination of the parents after consultation with the specialist.

In the more usual case, however, where one sex is identifiable as predominantly determined, corrective measures must be in the direction of the determined sex.

3. No one has the right, while actually (i.e., not because of mistaken sex identification) being a member of one sex, to attempt, by surgical or pharmacological alteration, to live as a member of the opposite sex. In the first place the

mutilations involved would be gravely illicit since they could in no way be defended under the principle of totality. Moreover, such alterations, for example, in a male who claims he has a "female mind" would not actually change his sex. He could not enter the state of matrimony as a female even if a plastic vagina had been constructed, for he remains actually a male. Nor could he marry a female, for he would now be impotent. In addition to all this, his transvestism would be an occasion of sin for himself and grave scandal for others.

General Procedures in Cases of Known or Suspected Impotence

Before Marriage: The doctor will see Catholic patients who are contemplating marriage and with whom there is some question of impotence. Depending on whether the patient is certainly impotent, or doubtfully impotent, or only temporarily impotent, the physician may safely follow one of the following norms:

If Impotence is Certain: If the patient contemplating marriage is certainly impotent it is within the scope of the doctor's duty to inform the patient of this, and even to indicate to the patient the impossibility of contracting a valid marriage.

If Impotence is Doubtful: When the doctor is not very certain that his patient is impotent, but has a positive reason for suspecting impotence, the doctor should first try to investigate and settle the doubt in his own mind, and then proceed as above if he becomes certain that impotence exists. If the doubt remains the physician should advise the patient to clear the matter through the ecclesiastical authorities.

If Impotence is Temporary: If impotence is present but can be corrected surgically or in some other legitimate way, and marriage is contemplated, although the canonical impediment does not exist in such a case, the patient does have an obligation either to have the condition corrected before the marriage, or to inform the proposed partner of the diffi-

culty with the intention of having it corrected after marriage.
The reason for this is that in handing over to the other
party the right to perfect copula, evidently one must take the
necessary means to permit the other party to exercise that
right, or to inform the other party if the right is to be temporarily suspended.

The doctor may inform the patient of this obligation, if
it seems prudent to do so in the individual case.

After Marriage: When the doctor discovers a case of impotence or suspected impotence after the couple have already been
through a marriage ceremony and have been living together as
man and wife, the situation becomes more difficult.

Consider the case of a woman with a vagina so small as to
preclude penetration by her putative husband, and yet who is
the mother of a child, conceived by semination at the labia and
delivered by caesarian section.

If Impotence is Doubtful: If the impotence is doubtful
and there is any hope of the couple performing perfect
copula, they may attempt marital intercourse until it is certain that it cannot be performed properly.

If Impotence is Certain: If the doctor discovers a supposedly married couple where impotence certainly exists,
without informing the parties of this fact, he should advise
them to consult their parish priest about the difficulties they
experience in trying to exercise their marital rights. The
doctor should not try to settle this case from a moral standpoint, but he would do well to tell the parties that if the
priest wishes to talk over the details of the problem with him,
he would be glad to do so.

If the impotence cannot be corrected, and the parties are
in good faith and do not know of the impediment, and if
separation is morally impossible; or if the priest believes that,
if told of the invalidity of their marriage, they will not separate and will thus be knowingly committing fornication, he
may leave them in good faith, in some cases.

If the impotence exists only in one party, and they do

separate, even though the marriage was invalid, the other
party is not free to remarry until after an ecclesiastical declaration of nullity. The same is true in cases of relative impotence under these circumstances.

Regarding the non-Catholic Patient: It will be noted that the
foregoing norms of the doctor-patient relationship have been
formulated envisioning a Catholic patient with an impotence
problem.

Even though impotence is an impediment of the natural law
and therefore the same for Catholics and non-Catholics alike—
the Church merely giving an authentic declaration of the natural
law in this matter—still the non-Catholic will normally not be in
a position to refer his problem to the ecclesiastical authorities.

In such cases, the doctor, bearing in mind the principle of
Canon 1068, that the impediment, in order to impede marriage,
must be certainly present, certainly perpetual, and certainly
antecedent to the marriage, should act according to the dictates
of his own prudent judgment, considering all the circumstances
of each individual case.

Other Impediments to Catholic Marriage

The impediment of impotence has been treated in great detail
because it is the one most likely to concern the doctor in his
practice. The other impediments to marriage will be treated only
by way of general information, and in their broad outlines.

Diriment Impediments: Aside from impotence, there are
other impediments which are also called "diriment" because
their effect, unless dispensed, is to invalidate marriage. Some of
these have the natural law or divine positive law as their source,
while others are purely canonical.

Age: A man can validly marry only after the age of sixteen,
and a woman can validly marry only after the age of fourteen,
which means the day after the sixteenth or the fourteenth birth-
day respectively. (Canon 1067).

The source of this impediment is ecclesiastical law, and it can
be dispensed. The natural law contains no impediment of age,

but in order to enter into a valid contract the parties must have the use of reason and at least a general knowledge of the meaning of the contract.

Ligamen: If one of the contracting parties is already bound by an existing valid marriage the diriment impediment of "ligamen" exists. (Canon 1069).

The impediment is of the natural law and the divine positive law, and cannot be dispensed. A civil divorce does not dissolve a previous marriage.

Disparity of Cult: The diriment impediment of disparity of cult exists between a non-baptized and one who has been baptized in the Catholic Church, or converted from heresy or schism to the Catholic Church, even if they have subsequently left the Church. (Canons 1070-1071).

Not only those who have been baptized by a priest, but also those who have been baptized by any other Catholic, as may occur in case of necessity, are "baptized in the Catholic Church." Thus a child of non-Catholic parents who was baptized by a Catholic doctor, in danger of death and then recovered, would seem to be subject to this impediment.[244]

The impediment, as diriment, is of ecclesiastical origin and can be dispensed.

Sacred Orders: Deacons, priests, and bishops cannot validly marry. The impediment is of ecclesiastical origin. It is never dispensed in the case of a bishop, but is sometimes dispensed in the case of a priest or a deacon. (Canon 1072).

Solemn Religious Profession: There is an ecclesiastical diriment impediment attached to the solemn vow of chastity, and in some cases even to the simple vow of chastity, in a religious order. These vows can be dispensed, and if they are dispensed the impediment ceases. (Canon 1073).

Violent Abduction or Detention: A man who, through physical violence, grave fear, fraud, or treachery abducts or detains a woman in order to marry her cannot do so validly until after she has been separated from him and freed from any influence exercised by him. (Canon 1074).

The impediment is of ecclesiastical law, and ceases with the cessation of the abduction or detention, together with the cessation of the influence of the abductor or detainer.

Crime: When one party is validly married, and then commits adultery with another, both knowing the validity of the aforementioned marriage, and they mutually:

1. either promise to marry;
2. or attempt marriage, even before a civil official;
3. or one of them kills, or has someone kill, the partner of the already existing marriage;
4. or even without the previously mentioned adultery both together conspire to kill and subsequently actually do kill the partner of the already existing marriage:

there exists between the two the diriment impediment of "crime," which is of ecclesiastical origin. (Canon 1075).

Consanguinity: The impediment of consanguinity invalidates marriage within the forbidden degrees of relationship. (Canon 1076).

The impediment is certainly diriment from the natural law between parent and child, and probably diriment from natural law between grandparent and grandchild, and between brother and sister.

The ecclesiastical diriment impediment exists between all in the direct line of descent, and up to second cousins inclusive in the collateral line.

The impediment of consanguinity, in so far as it is purely ecclesiastical, can be dispensed. It cannot be dispensed in those cases mentioned above which are either certainly or probably of the natural law.

Affinity: Affinity is relationship by marriage and exists between a husband and the blood relatives of his wife, and between a wife and the blood relatives of her husband.

Affinity is a diriment impediment of purely ecclesiastical law and extends indefinitely in the direct line but only to first cousins by marriage inclusively in the collateral line. (Canon 1077).

There are many complicated and involved cases concerning affinity and consanguinity which will not be discussed here.

Spiritual Relationship: A diriment impediment of ecclesiastical law arises between a baptized person and the one who baptized him, as well as between a baptized person and his god-father and godmother. The impediment is of purely ecclesiastical origin and is readily dispensed. (Canon 1079).

Legal Relationship: This is an impediment found in the civil law of some countries, which arises from legal adoption. Canon law, in this unique case, merely "canonizes" the civil law, i.e., makes the civil impediment canonical. The impediment does not exist anywhere in the United States. (Canon 1080).

Merely Prohibiting Impediments

The only two additional impediments which need to be mentioned here are merely prohibiting impediments, that is, they make a marriage illicit, but not invalid.

Simple Vow: A simple vow which is directly opposed to marriage, such as a vow not to marry; or one that is indirectly opposed to marriage, in so far as marriage would make the observance of the vow very difficult, or render its fulfillment impossible, such as a simple vow of chastity or virginity, or a vow to receive sacred orders or to enter religion, render marriage illicit until the vow is dispensed. (Canon 1058).

Mixed Religion: This is a merely prohibiting impediment which exists between two baptized, one of whom is a member of the Catholic Church while the other is a member of an heretical, schismatic, or atheistic sect. The impediment is of ecclesiastical origin and can be dispensed. (Canon 1064).

Medico-Moral Aspects of Marriage

In the previous pages we have treated, in some detail, certain of the canonical aspects of marriage which are most likely to become the concern of the physician. After thus investigating the nature of the marriage contract, in its canonical implications, it is necessary to look at some of the moral implications of the contract. At times the doctor will find himself in a position of peculiar advantage for giving some word of direction along these lines.

It will be recalled that the natural law contract of marriage, when entered into by two baptized individuals, is a sacrament. A sacrament is defined as an outward sign, instituted by Christ, to confer grace. The outward sign is the matrimonial contract itself, which is represented by Saint Paul as symbolizing the union between Christ and His Church. And like this intimate and sanctifying union, marriage too sanctifies the parties of the contract and produces in their souls a deeper radiation of their participation in the divine life which we call sanctifying grace.

With this background in mind, the physician should be aware of his opportunity to direct married couples, and more especially those about to be married, along the lines of correct thinking in regard to the broad outlines of their state of life.

Because of the unfavorable circumstances in which too many first learn "the facts of life," many patients will be found to bear the scars of psychic trauma in this regard.

In consultation with such patients it is of paramount importance to approach the sacrament of matrimony on a supernatural level in terms of a beautiful and intimate union of body and soul, explaining conjugal love and human generation as instituted and blessed by God: a reflection of the inner life of the blessed Trinity and a symbol of the sanctifying and cleansing union between Christ and His Church.

What might be called the "birds and bees approach" to this matter, even for the very young, is shallow, incomplete, and degrading to the very nature of the subject matter.

In his consultation with those about to be married, the physician can do a great deal toward insuring a holy and happy married life. Regarding the approach to marital intimacy in the beginning of marriage, gentleness and consideration of the other party should be advised.

It will sometimes help to produce a proper mental attitude if the doctor points out that any virtue is the proper ordering of human actions; and that when a man and wife by their marital relations grow in holiness of life and supernaturally merit precisely in the virtue of purity.

The physician, by his own attitude and manner of speaking, can help the young couple to advance to the point where their physical union becomes more and more an approach to that deeper union of mind and heart and life which should always be the crowning glory of this sacramental state of life.

Family Planning and Fertility Control

From the middle of the present century the insistent concern of demographers with the problem of projected population increases beyond the resources of civilization has led to an exigent anxiety regarding fertility control.

Even before this, in the first quarter of the century, the traditional Judaico-Christian ethic of the uncompromised marital act had been gradually modified outside the Catholic Church, as can be seen most vividly by comparing the moral directives of the Lambeth Conferences of the Anglican Church of 1920, 1930 and 1958. The 1920 Lambeth Conference repeated the absolute condemnation of contraception in the strongest possible terms, and called for a vigorous campaign against the open or secret sale of contraceptives. The 1930 Conference again affirmed that the procreation of children was the primary purpose of marriage, but conceded that in certain limited circumstances contraception might be morally acceptable, and the 1958 Conference endorsed birth control as a responsibility laid by God on parents everywhere. In somewhat similar terms the General Board of the National Council of Churches, in February 1961, endorsed the use of birth control devices as part of Christian responsibility in family planning.

Meanwhile the Catholic Church, sensitive to these changes and with her own sharp self-image and firm doctrinal stability, condemned this weakening of the moral context of marriage and in December of 1930, solemnly reasserted the traditional doctrine in the following words of Pope Pius XI's Encyclical on Christian Marriage:

> But no reason, however grave, may be put forward by which anything intrinsically against nature may become conformable to nature and morally good. Since, therefore, the conjugal act is destined primarily by nature for the begetting of children, those who in exercising it deliberately frustrate

its natural power and purpose sin against nature and commit a deed which is shameful and intrinsically vicious.

Since, therefore, openly departing from the uninterrupted Christian tradition, some recently have judged it possible solemnly to declare another doctrine regarding this question, the Catholic Church, to whom God has entrusted the defense of the integrity and purity of morals, standing erect in the midst of the moral ruin which surrounds her in order that she may preserve the chastity of the nuptial union from being defiled by this foul stain, raises her voice in token of Divine ambassadorship and through Our mouth proclaims anew: any use whatsoever of matrimony exercised in such a way that the act is deliberately frustrated in its natural power to generate life is an offense against the law of God and of nature, and those who indulge in such are branded with the guilt of a grave sin.[245]

Subsequently, as the moral doctrine regarding contraceptive practice continued to be modified in the Protestant theologies, Pope Pius XII reviewed again, in detail, the Catholic doctrine in his now famous Allocution to the Association of Italian Midwives (October 28, 1951). In this allocution the Pope recalled the fundamental moral acceptability of periodic continence (the "rhythm method" of family planning) and treated, in considerable detail, the circumstances under which it is appropriately used. At the same time he reasserted the Church's condemnation of direct contraception and reaffirmed the teaching of Pius XI's Encyclical on Christian Marriage precisely in these words: "any attempt on the part of the husband and wife to deprive this act (conjugal intercourse) of its inherent force or to impede the procreation of a new life, either in the performance of the act itself, or in the course of the development of its natural consequences, is immoral."[246] On the same occasion Pope Pius XII also declared that: "direct sterilization—that is, sterilization which aims, either as a means or as an end in itself, to render childbearing impossible—is a grave violation of the moral law," and he explicitly applied this to either permanent or temporary sterilization.

It is likewise interesting to note that, even at this time, the

Pontiff dealt explicitly and extensively with the modern personalistic approach to the marital act and the presumed impossibility of prolonged abstinence. Indicating the truths to be found in these concepts, and the errors that lie in their exaggerations, he warned against a too biological approach to the mystique of married love.

Subsequently, in December 1965, the Second Vatican Council enunciated the fundamental doctrine of the Catholic Church regarding fertility control in the following words:

> Therefore when there is question of harmonizing conjugal love with the responsible transmission of life, the moral aspect of any procedure does not depend solely on sincere intentions or on an evaluation of motives. It must be determined by objective standards. These, based on the nature of the human person and his acts, preserve the full sense of mutual self-giving and human procreation in the context of true love. Such a goal cannot be achieved unless the virtue of conjugal chastity is sincerely practiced. Relying on these principles, sons of the Church may not undertake methods of regulating procreation which are found blameworthy by the teaching authority of the Church in its unfolding of the divine law.

To this paragraph the Council Fathers attached "Footnote 14," in which reference is made to the Encyclical of Pius XI on Christian Marriage and the allocution of Pius XII to the Association of Italian Midwives. The Council, in this same footnote, likewise made reference to an address of Pope Paul VI to a group of Cardinals (June 23, 1964) in which he declared that the steroid approach to fertility control was under study, but that in the meantime the condemnation of the use of the progestational steroids for contraceptive purposes, as enunciated by Pope Pius XII in an address to a meeting of hematologists (September 12, 1958), was to be observed. The Council then concluded footnote 14 with the following words: "Certain questions which need further and more careful investigation have been handed over, at the command of the Supreme Pontiff, to a commission for the study of population, family, and births, in order that, after it fulfills its functions, the Supreme Pontiff may pass judgment. With the doctrine of the magisterium in this state, this holy Synod does not intend to propose immediate concrete solutions."[247]

Thus the Fathers of Vatican II left the matter of certain details of positive contraception to be re-examined and studied more deeply, and placed the final decision in the hands of the Roman Pontiff. That decision was finally presented to the entire Church on July 25, 1968 by Pope Paul VI in his encyclical *Humanae Vitae* on the transmission of human life.

Stressing again the dignity and exalted characteristics of conjugal love and the sacredness of marriage, as well as the exigencies of responsible parenthood, the Pope reiterated and reconfirmed the traditional teaching of the Catholic Church on contraception—that: "each and every marriage act must remain open to the transmission of life."[248] While the document does not go into a detailed treatment of various contraceptive practices, but is much more taken up with the positive values of marriage, the Pope did reiterate certain aspects of the Church's teaching with regard to sterilization as follows: "Equally to be excluded, as the teaching authority of the Church has frequently declared, is direct sterilization, whether perpetual or temporary, whether of the man or of the woman. Similarly excluded is every action which, either in anticipation of the conjugal act, or in its accomplishment, or in the development of its natural consequences, proposes, whether as an end or as a means, to render procreation impossible."

Thus it is evident that although the encyclical presented a comprehensive moral condemnation of contraceptive practices, its purpose was not only to reiterate the traditional teaching of the Catholic Church in this regard, but likewise to formally extend that teaching to the more recent questions of pharmacological fertility control.

Contraceptive Medication: The usual directly contraceptive instruments and compounds are designed to thwart the purpose of the act of intercourse either by placing an artificial barrier between the sperm and the ovum, by using some extrinsic device such as a condom or occlusive pessary; or by destroying the viability of the spermatozoa with spermicidal douches or jellies.

Recently there has been considerable investigation into a more physiological approach to contraception by means of pharmacologically induced temporary sterilization, which is brought about by the suppression or modification of the endocrine processes essential to reproduction.

Recalling the delicately balanced complexity of nerve responses, regulatory hormones, sex-hormones, enzymes, other endocrine mechanisms and still unexplored biological processes upon which the production and effective union of ovum and sperm depends, it is not difficult to see how pharmacologically induced alterations in these patterns could result in temporary sterility through producing a physiologic pattern hostile to ovulation.

Sieve's report, in 1952, on regulated doses of phosphorylated hesperidin counteracting the enzyme reaction whereby the sperm penetrates the zona pellucida of the ovum gave rise to a rash of "contraceptive pill" articles in the popular press.[249] Although the effectiveness of this approach to contraception was later called into question, investigation into various progestational compounds as ovulation inhibitors advanced rapidly. Research in this latter area had not been primarily oriented around contraceptive procedures, but had been applied rather to the use of synthetic progestational compounds as tests for ovarian function, correction of menstrual disorders, and the preservation of pregnancies in habitual abortors. Moreover, even the direct suppression of ovulation may be of therapeutic value in treating severe cases of dysmenorrhea and endometriosis. The same compounds, however, are effective in the suppression of ovulation as a directly contraceptive procedure, and this aspect of the investigation had not gone unnoticed. Moreover, similar compounds designed to inhibit spermatogenesis in the male have been likewise investigated with success. The moral evaluation which follows applies, *mutatis mutandis*, equally to suppression of ovulation and inhibition of spermatogenesis.

Moral Comment: Because this new pharmacological approach to contraception is achieved by alteration of the body mechanism prior to coitus, and leaves the act of intercourse apparently natural and normal, some had questioned whether or not it might be a legitimate method of birth control.

When such medication is taken with directly contraceptive intent it is clearly a method of direct, although temporary, sterilization. As such, it is in direct conflict with the teaching of the Roman Pontiffs condemning all direct sterilization.

Frequently these medications are used as truly therapeutic agents to correct physiologic and functional abnormalities of the generative system. In such cases if the concomitant temporary sterility results, it is, in the moral order, rather a side-effect, foreseen but not sought, and the morality of the therapy is to be evaluated under the principle of double effect. Such, for example, would be the use of the progestational compounds for the relief of abnormal menstrual bleeding, to correct other pathologic conditions brought on by endocrine imbalance, or to correct irregularities in the ovulation-menstruation cycle.

In any of the situations where the principle of double effect properly applies to the temporary sterility resulting from this type of therapy, husband and wife need not abstain from their marital relations during the periods of sterility.

It might be noted that the application of the principle of double effect to their therapeutic use may become more complex because of harmful side effects of the medications. There has been question of a carcinogenic potential in the use of some of these compounds.[250] There is also serious question regarding the safety of the compounds in the presence of hypertensive, vascular or neurologic diseases, among others.[251] Moreover as the continued use of such compounds builds up a clinical history, the list of suspected or identified complications and dangerous side-effects constantly grows longer.

Aside from such deleterious side effects which have not yet been fully evaluated, there is no moral contraindication to the therapy as a means to establish a more regular and normal ovulation cycle. This can be particularly advantageous in the practice of periodic continence.

When the presence of irregular ovulation arises from hormone imbalance, it should be remembered that the hypophysis (of the brain), the ovary, the uterine lining, and the hormonal balance of the blood stream are all part of the ovulatory-menstrual mechanism. This whole mechanism, as pathologically irregular, is now to be viewed under the principle of totality.

The progestational approach is to alter the hormone imbalance in the blood stream as a means (hopefully) to restore the hormone balance. There has been clinical indication that this therapy will be effective in some cases. The concomitant temporary inhibition of ovulation can be justified under the principle of double effect.

Another laudable therapeutic use of the progestational compounds is the attempt to correct maternal hormone imbalance during pregnancy in an effort to forestall spontaneous abortion. It should be noted, however, that while no untoward effects on the fetus have been clearly attributable to natural progesterone, Lawson Wilkins, M.D., has reported several cases of masculinization of female fetuses after the use of synthetic hormones with sufficient androgenic action to orient the development of the sensitive female fetus toward pseudo-hermaphrodism. Moralists would agree with Dr. Wilkin's comment regarding the use of such compounds in the prevention of spontaneous abortion: "If they are valuable and necessary, the ones which are least likely to cause fetal masculinization should be used."²⁵²

Other Contraceptive Techniques: In the following pages certain common methods of contraception are discussed briefly. The moral aspects of their use is viewed in the light of the Catholic doctrine outlined above.

The "withdrawal" of the male partner prior to ejaculation is a seriously immoral distortion of the marital act. It is likewise liable to be contraceptively ineffective because of the likelihood of seminal distillation before withdrawal as well as the inability to time the moment of withdrawal. The practice is likewise open to the danger of psychogenic impotence in the male and frigidity in the female.

The commercially available condom is a close-fitting sheath for the penis, usually made of rubber, latex, or the cacea of sheep. It is the most widely used and least clinically controlled mechanical contraceptive available. Although its quality is subject to the supervision of the Food and Drug Administration, the major cause of contraceptive failure is said to be rupture of the sheath during coitus.

It is the teaching of the Catholic Church that the use of the condom as a measure of fertility control is an essential distortion of the marital act and is always immoral.

A thin rubber dome, or diaphragm, encircled by a spring-ring, to cover the area from the fornix behind the cervix to the pubic arch, blocks the cervix to the passage of the male ejaculate and holds accessory spermicidal cream or jelly against the cervix. After intercourse the male ejaculate is expelled from the vagina by simply bearing down. This mechanical blocking and rejection of the male ejaculate is considered, in Catholic teaching, to be an unnatural and immoral distortion of the marital act.

Jellies, Creams, and Foams:

These are pharmacological spermicidal agents introduced into the vagina prior to intercourse which are designed to prevent conception by the destruction of the male spermatozoa. Although this contraceptive approach may seem to leave the marital act itself undistorted, its morality differs little from that of the diaphragm or the cervical cap method. Catholic teaching views this contraceptive destruction of the spermatozoa in the marital act itself as seriously disordered and morally wrong.

In the late 1920's E. Grafenberg, a German physician, popularized the notion of a thin indwelling intrauterine silver wire as a contraceptive device. Because its use was associated with inflammatory irritation, the Grafenberg ring never became popular. Subsequent modifications in design and materials have resulted in a resurgence of various intrauterine devices made of silk worm gut, stainless steel springs, and various plastic coils, rings, loops and spirals. They are neither completely protective nor entirely free from undesirable and even extremely serious complications, not the least of which is uterine perforation.[253]

Not the least of the moral problems presented by the intrauterine device is the distinct possibility that its mode of action may not actually be prevention of conception (although this may occur at times) but rather prevention of the implantation of the conceived embryo. Thus, although not technically (in the clinical sense) an abortifacient (since the medical definition of abortion includes the notion of accomplished implantation) it would nonetheless involve the same moral malice as abortion in the destruction of the non-viable conceptus. As late as 1965 a joint study by the Departments of Obstetrics of the University of Pennsylvania and the University of Michigan made the following report.

"Women wearing intrauterine devices do ovulate and can conceive. The fertilized ovum may fail to implant because it reaches the uterus before its invasive ability is fully developed or before endometrial changes have advanced enough to receive it. There also is the possibility, however, that an intrauterine device can alter stromal development enough to make it unsuitable for implantation."[254] This question alone is sufficient to reject the intrauterine devices on moral grounds, nor would they be acceptable in the context of Catholic doctrine even apart from this consideration.

The "morning-after" Approach

The so-called morning-after approach to conception control demands very careful moral consideration because the same semantic confusion as mentioned in regard to the use of the intrauterine device has likewise beclouded this issue to a considerable degree. It will be recalled that the theological concept of *abortion* extends to the destruction of a newly conceived life from the moment of conception to viability, whereas the accepted medical use of the term "abortion" is usually applied only to the destruction of the unborn life *after* implantation of the embryo on the uterine wall and before viability. Thus, in the embryonic life span, there is an initial period of quite some days (the time span between conception in the upper quadrant of the fallopian tube and subsequent implantation of the embryo on the wall of the uterus) during which the destruction of the new life is theologically identified with the moral malice of abortion, but in medical circles is illogically called contraception (illogically in the sense that conception has already occurred and thus the destructive move is not "contra-conception" but rather "contra-conceptus").

Thus, within the medical armamentarium, the use of large doses of diethylstilbestrol (DES) when there is suspicion of contraceptive failure, or the common practice of dilation and curettage (D and C) after rape present the moral malice, not of contraception, but of abortion. Indeed this problem, precisely as it relates to treatment after rape, is explicitly noted in the current (1971) edition of the *Ethical and Religious Directives for Catholic Health Facilities* as follows: "It is to be noted that curettage of the endometrium after rape to prevent implantation of a possible embryo is morally equivalent to abortion." (Directive 24).

Moreover it should be noted that, in addition to the fact that this embryo-destruction sequence is evident in the morning-after approach, it has not been completely excluded (by scientific studies) as a possible mechanism even in the use of some of those contraceptive medications whose primary action is designed to inhibit ovulation.

Trichomonas Vaginitis: Trichomonas is a genus of parasitic flagellate protozoa which occurs in a variety of forms and in various tissues. A species (trichomonas vaginalis) infects the female at the vagina, especially in the presence of acid secretion. Occurring at some time in about twenty per cent of the female population, it produces a refractory vaginal discharge which is foaming and malodorous and which is accompanied by minute hemorrhages of the mucosa. Edema, burning and itching of the vulva are present. Both urination and intercourse become difficult and painful.

The condition is persistent and difficult to eradicate. Various vaginal suppositories, powders, and medicinal jellies are prescribed and at least one oral tablet has been tried.

A moral question arises from the conviction in medical circles that a large percentage of these infections probably result from the parasite being transmitted by the male organ during intercourse. Hence many physicians advise the use of a condom during intercourse while treatment is in progress. This practice is clearly immoral. It cannot be justified under the principle of double effect (as though intending only the prophylaxis and merely permitting the contraceptive effect) because the very act of condomistic intercourse is an exercise of the generative function in such a way that conception is artificially blocked. This is, in itself, contrary to the natural law.

More recently investigative studies of various chemotherapeutic agents have given great promise of a solution to this difficult problem, but frequently the condom technique is continued.

Morality of Marital Intercourse in Particular Circumstances

Although the doctor should not be expected to supply the place of the moral theologian in marriage guidance, the following points of moral theology should be studied carefully. A clear knowledge of these points will be very important for giving the proper advice and direction to some patients.

Intercourse during Times of Temporary Sterility : For a husband and wife to have marital relations at a time when conception cannot take place, even though their only explicit intention for doing so is the enjoyment of their marital relations, presents no moral problem.

These acts of intercourse foster mutual love and devotion, solidify and foster that atmosphere of a devoted family life in which it is proper for present or future children to be raised, and such acts are at least implicitly referred to this end.

The Practice of Periodic Continence : The question treated immediately above, namely, the morality of marital intercourse during periods of temporary sterility, is not quite the same as the question of positively limiting intercourse to non-ovulation periods precisely in order to avoid conception.

This practice is referred to as "periodic continence" or "rhythm" and consists in limiting marital intercourse to those periods during the menstrual cycle when ovulation, and hence conception, is least likely to take place.

Note carefully, as stated above and for the reasons already explained, there is nothing morally wrong with having intercourse during these periods of sterility. The only moral consideration arises under the aspect of limiting intercourse to the periodic naturally sterile times.

Pius XII: "If the carrying out of this theory means nothing more than that the couple can make use of their matrimonial rights on the days of natural sterility too, there is nothing against it, for in so doing they neither hinder nor injure in any way the consummation of the natural act and its further natural consequences."[255]

The morality of limiting marital intercourse to the sterile periods is summed up in the following points, drawn from the papal documents:

1. The married state does include the design of the natural law and the divine positive law for the conservation of the human race.
2. Couples who exercise their marital rights continuously have an obligation to at least sometimes be willing to accept their share of this duty: of assisting, if they can, in the conservation of the race.
3. However, since there is question here of an affirmative precept of law, there are excusing causes.

The papal pronouncements do not indicate how many children a married couple should have in order to fulfill the obligation of their state of life. Certainly there is no indication that married people must have as many children as they are physically and economically capable of having.

Neither do the papal pronouncements delineate how serious a reason is required to hold oneself excused from the obligation of accepting the duties of procreation, or at least of not side-stepping them, or for how long a time; except that (as Pius XII pointed out) to do so always, or for "a very long time," without serious reason, would be morally wrong.

But, since it is clearly stated that serious medical, eugenic, economic, or social reasons can excuse from the obligation for a very long time, or even for the whole of married life, it would seem to follow that less serious reasons would excuse for a less prolonged time.

Considerations such as illness in the family, inadequate housing, the necessity of the mother to work, economic insecurity for the future, military service and similar circumstances could be sufficient reasons for practicing periodic continence for a shorter or longer time, depending on how long the circumstances are verified.

Moreover, those couples who have already had several children would certainly not seem to be guilty of sin even if they practiced rhythm for a long time without serious reason, or for at least a reasonable cause.

In addition to the consideration of the sufficient reason for the practice of periodic continence, there are two additional questions which must be answered in the affirmative before a couple can undertake this practice without blame. These questions are: "Are the parties *willing*—and are they *able*, to practice periodic continence?"

The question of mutual willingness to practice rhythm arises out of the grave obligation incumbent upon each partner to accede to the reasonable and serious request for marital relations, unless by mutual agreement the act is postponed.

Theologians commonly teach that a spouse has the right temporarily to refuse intercourse when the partner has committed adultery or other sex crime, or is guilty of onanistic approaches to the marital act. Drunkenness and insanity are also reasons for refusing intercourse, as is legitimate separation with ecclesiastical approval. Moreover, excusing causes for postponing intercourse are identified in any serious danger or inconvenience to one of the parties, such as might arise out of physical debility, danger of contagion, immoderate frequency of the act, etc.

This problem would arise only when the sterile periods are being observed for a reason not sufficiently serious in itself to excuse from the obligation of rendering the marital debitum, such as circumstances seriously affecting the health or welfare of either party, or of the offspring.

In addition to mutual willingness to engage in the practice of periodic continence, there arises the question of the ability to do so without the parties placing themselves in a proximate occasion of sin. Can the parties continue the fostering of their mutual love and harmonious affections for one another under these circumstances and still safeguard their marital chastity? Can the possible temptations to solitary sexual activity be rendered remote and be controlled? These questions must be answered in the affirmative before a couple can properly adopt the practice of periodic continence.

In consultation with the Catholic patient regarding the use of rhythm the doctor should decide on the seriousness of the medical indication for its use and so -inform the patient, meanwhile suggesting that the patient talk the matter over with the confessor.

Note that in these cases the couple is seeking *advice* and *direction* regarding the moral dimension of the use of periodic continence in their particular circumstances. One occasionally hears of Catholics "seeking *permission* of their confessor to practice rhythm"—a turn of phrase as distasteful as it is erroneous.

The doctor need not hesitate to offer advice or assistance with regard to the use of rhythm, when such advice or assistance is sought. Nor is the physician obliged to assure himself that the patient has a sufficient reason for using rhythm.

It has been frequently charged that the Catholic Church is somehow inconsistent in her doctrine of responsible parenthood by condemning positive contraception but permitting the use of periodic continence since, as the objection usually states, the results are the same. This charge arises from pragmatic feeling rather than from theological speculation. The moral deformity of positive contraception does not lie precisely in the intention to avoid conception, or in the desire not to have a child at this time, but in the way in which this intention and desire is implemented. Pope Paul VI treats this dimension of the question in *Humanae Vitae* as follows:

The Church is coherent with herself when she considers recourse to the infecund periods to be licit, while at the same time condemning, as being always illicit, the use of means directly contrary to fecundation, even if such use is inspired by reasons which may appear honest and serious. In reality, there are essential differences between the two cases; in the former, the married couple make legitimate use of a natural disposition; in the latter, they impede the development of natural processes. It is true that, in the one and the other case, the married couple are concordant in the positive will of avoiding children for plausible reasons, seeking the certainty that offspring will not arrive; but it is also true that only in the former case are they able to renounce the use of marriage in the fecund periods when, for just motives, procreation is not desirable, while making use of it during infecund periods to manifest their affection and to safeguard their mutual fidelity. By so doing, they give proof of a truly and integrally honest love.

For those who are observing periodic continence under the proper circumstances, there is no moral objection to using accepted aids (e.g., basal temperature charts, etc.) for identifying the onset of ovulation.

Permanent Sterility : Permanent sterility, (as distinct from impotence), even if due to absence of part of the generative system, does not render intercourse illicit. The only exception to this norm is had when one of the parties submits to a sterilizing operation, with contraceptive intent.

An example of this would be contraceptive bilateral tubal ligation or vasectomy. Marital intercourse is wrong for such individuals until after sincere repentance, simply because their contraceptive distortion of the meaning of the marriage act continues in their use of marriage. If the contraceptively induced condition can be repaired without serious suffering or risk the repentance could hardly be called sincere until such repair is undertaken.

As long as the development of surgical technique for such an anastomosis remains limited to a doubtfully successful surgical

result, however, it would be difficult to identify an obligation
to undergo the surgery.

Surgical Anastomosis of Vas Deferens: O'Connor's classical
paper on this subject in 1948 publicized the fact that successful
surgical anastomosis had been achieved in a number of cases.[256]

A review of the literature on the subject indicates that the
perfection of the technique and the success of the procedure
have advanced steadily since that time. Only four years after
O'Connor's paper, Dorsey read a paper at the Western Section
of the American Urological Association in which he said:

> The majority of the medical profession, and a surprising
> number of urologists, are of the opinion that bilateral vasec-
> tomy produces a state of irreversible sterility. O'Connor in
> 1948 stated that out of 750 urologists who had returned his
> questionnaire, 615 had never attempted surgical reunion of
> the vas deferens. It is the purpose of this paper to demon-
> strate that anastomosis of the vas deferens, or vasorrhapy, is
> successful in a sufficiently large percentage of cases as to
> justify its more frequent performance.[257]

Subsequently, Stanwood Schmidt could go so far as to say
that surgical anastomosis of the vas deferens after purposeful
vasectomy is an operation which can be performed successfully
in the *vast majority of cases.*[258]

It should, of course, be pointed out that the anatomical site
of the vasectomy or occlusion has a great deal to do with the
predictability of success in these operations.

These advances in surgical technique raise several questions.
What obligation is there for a man who is conscious of bilateral
nodular occlusion of the vas deferens to seek surgical restoration
of the *lumen* before attempting marriage; and secondly, what
obligation does the male partner to a valid marriage have to
seek surgical correction for purposefully induced sterility by
ligation of the vas deferens?

In spite of the surgical advances in this regard and in view
of the persisting "tongue-in-cheek" attitude of so many physicians as to the chance of successfully restoring potency of the

lumen, we believe that, although surgical correction should be encouraged, the general obligation to submit to it cannot be pressed at this time.

Canonical Impotence: Canonical impotence, incurred subsequent to a valid marriage, e.g., after therapeutic castration of the male partner, does not dissolve the marriage. Nor does it render intercourse illicit as long as the parties are still capable of the marital act.

But if they are no longer capable of intercourse, they may still venereally enjoy the other intimacies permitted to married people so long as these do not induce orgasm in either partner.[259] Such an orgasm, willfully induced outside of an act of marital intercourse, would simply be masturbation.

However, a situation sometimes comes about subsequent to a valid marriage and due to the female partner's condition wherein perfect copula is either physically impossible or extremely painful. In such cases semination may be possible only at the entrance to the vagina. If such is the case such limited intercourse may be morally permitted.[260]

Complications of Senility: Likewise marital intercourse is permitted to those married people who, because of old age or some illness, frequently seminate outside the vagina of their spouse, as long as there is some hope of performing the act properly.

Marital Relations during Pregnancy: During pregnancy it is obviously wrong for married people to have intercourse at such times as it would constitute some real risk of abortion. It is the prerogative of the doctor to decide on the time and extent of such risk.

Marital Relations during Puerperium: Married people should abstain from their marital relations during that part of the puerperium in which the doctor judges that intercourse would involve some risk to the wife.

If Danger is Associated with Future Pregnancy: Women who have been advised by a doctor that they may die if they become pregnant again and attempt to bring forth another child are not, for this reason, forbidden to have intercourse. Experience shows both that such predictions are frequently false and that these dangers are often over-stressed by many doctors. Moreover, the danger connected with the actual intercourse is quite remote since conception and the development of the fetus is so uncertain. The danger, however, should be rendered even more remote by the observance of periodic continence.

Even in these cases, however, the use of contraceptives or contraceptive sterilization, although clinically indicated from a medical viewpoint, remains contrary to the teaching of the Catholic Church. It must be remembered that the Church teaches that all contraceptive intercourse is a basic distortion of conjugal love and not to be admitted even for clinical considerations so serious as to demand temporary or even total abstinence from marital intercourse. This obviously entails great mutual sacrifice for the good of the beloved—a notion neither foreign to nor destructive of genuine love. It is not surprising, of course, that many people simply reject this teaching. A deep and sincere faith is needed to pit the wisdom of the Church against clinical contraception in our contraceptively oriented culture. .

Defective Offspring Usually Anticipated: Married people who have good reason to believe that spontaneous abortion will follow conception, or that if the pregnancy runs its course the child will be abnormal, cannot for this reason be obliged to abstain from intercourse, but neither is contraception nor abortion permissible under these circumstances. Here one must consider the fundamental right of the spouses to their marital intercourse, plus the uncertainty of conception in a particular marital act; plus the fact that, if conception takes place, no real injustice is inflicted upon the new life. Theologians teach that the infant will at least enjoy an eternal state of natural beatitude. In some cases, however, the couple might be prudently advised to practice periodic continence.

Cooperation in Marital Intercourse

Without undertaking the moral direction of his patient, the doctor should study and understand the following cases of cooperation in marital intercourse as a necessary background for instructing or advising his patients.

Although, in the doctrine of the Catholic Church, the moral disorder of contraceptive intercourse is evident when both partners are party to the contraceptive intent and practice, some variation of the moral assessment is necessarily introduced when only one of the spouses is determined in contraceptive intent. Because of the nature and importance of the marital relationship, problems of cooperation and the limitations of responsibility arise in the presence of a conscientious disapproval of the contraceptive practice of the partner together with the deep human exigency for the use of marriage.

The only absolute moral dilemma in this matter is in the circumstance of the husband using a condom sheath. Such an act of pseudo-intercourse is, objectively and from the very beginning of the act, not marital intercourse at all, but rather an artificial distortion of it. The only possible answer on the part of the wife is absolute refusal or, under physical duress, simple passivity.

If, on the other hand, the husband interrupts the natural coitus by withdrawal before insemination and his wife has done all that she reasonably can to dissuade him from this practice, her participation in the act is morally acceptable, both from the viewpoint of her own intention and from the nature of the act itself, up until the moment of withdrawal. Here, as in the following cases, her sincere attempt to dissuade him from this practice balances her obligation in charity to try to correct his moral wrong-doing. Under these circumstances she may participate in this use of marriage as long as it remains a marital act provided she is free of contraceptive intent. She may do this either in response to her husband's invitation or on her own initiative, and she may likewise prepare herself to experience orgasm while their union remains integral and enjoy the spontaneous (but not artificially induced) fulfillment of its sequelae.[261]

Under the same moral principles, the integrity of a partner's marital intercourse with a spouse who has achieved pharmacological (or surgical) sterilization contrary to the will of the other, is evident. The non-contraceptive partner has, after all, the radical right to marital intercourse and the material cooperation in the wrong-doing of the spouse is defensible, particularly in view of the fact that the entire act of intercourse itself remains integral. The partner cannot honestly either encourage or approve the contraceptive practice of the spouse, and indeed must honestly try to dissuade from it, but neither is the partner obliged to abstain from the use of marriage because of it.

While the same view can be defended in favor of the husband whose wife uses an occlusive diaphragm, it is our opinion that the presence of an intrauterine device precludes cooperation of the husband in a marital act which might result in conception and the subsequent destruction of the conceptus.

A Word of Caution: The foregoing comments on cooperation in onanistic intercourse are put here in order that the doctor may have a fuller general background for dealing with patients beset by these problems. In every instance, however, there will be elements to be considered which will demand that the final answer to such problems be left in the hands of a trained moral theologian.

In much the same way as the general practitioner should have a sufficient knowledge of the more complicated diseases to enable him to diagnose and refer his patient to a specialist, so here the doctor should not do more than diagnose such a situation and send his Catholic patient for further spiritual direction. Before advising a non-Catholic patient in these matters the doctor himself would do well to consult a theologian on the details of the individual case.

Finally, it should be evident that a physician who, because of his religious beliefs or philosophical convictions, rejects positive contraception as immoral, cannot advise or prescribe the use of contraceptives and still maintain his own personal integrity and intellectual honesty in the matter.

The Morality of Sterility Tests

Certain moral problems related to marriage and with a direct bearing on the practice of medicine arise in connection with tests designed to supply desired information in problems of sterility.

The procedures generally employed in testing females for sterility do not constitute any real moral problem. The only word of caution is medical as well as moral, and consists in the admonition that methods which introduce foreign substances into the peritoneal cavity by way of the fallopian tubes, such as is done in certain forms of salpingography, should be undertaken only by one well versed in these procedures, due to the danger which they constitute in inexperienced hands.

The moral problems involved in testing the male for sterility can be reduced to the morality of the various methods employed for collecting sperm for examination.

Masturbation and Onanism: Masturbation may be defined as the complete exercise of the generative function outside of marriage, or at least apart from the marriage act; or in such a way, even in an act of intercourse, that the generation of offspring is excluded in some positive way. This latter is properly called onanism.

Both masturbation and onanism have been indicated by some physicians as the preferable methods of obtaining sperm samples for examination.

Moral Aspect: Both masturbation and onanism are intrinsically wrong and no purpose, however good, can make them right. Therefore, masturbation, intercourse with an integral condom, or intercourse modified by withdrawal before ejaculation, in order to collect sperm for examination, are always under all circumstances contrary to Catholic teaching.

Pius XI: "Any use of matrimony whatsoever in the exercise of which the act is deprived, by human interference, of its natural power to procreate life, is an offense against the law of God and nature, and those who commit it are guilty of grave sin."

Moreover it might be pointed out here that in 1929 the Holy Office was asked if masturbation could be permitted to obtain sperm for examination as a diagnostic procedure. The reply of the Holy Office was an explicit condemnation of the practice.

It is obvious, of course, that masturbation is clinically the most convenient method for obtaining sperm for examination, and it is true that some recent theologians have rejected the Church's teaching in this matter. Their opinions, however, cannot command the respect of the faithful, nor can they be viewed as "solidly probable" for the following reasons: (1) The prohibition of masturbation follows from the basic Catholic teaching on human sexuality and the dissident writers supply no adequate theological explanation defending their different stand on clinical masturbation. Indeed many of them simply reject the basic Catholic teaching on human sexuality. (2) Official Catholic teaching has in no way indicated that the clinical setting provides an exception to the ordinary teaching on masturbation. (3) The traditional teaching was reaffirmed by the Bishops of the United States in their approval of *The Ethical and Religious Directives for Catholic Health Facilities* in November 1971. (cf. Directive 21).

Aspiration and Prostate Massage: The aspiration of seminal fluid from the testes or the epididymis by means of a needle and syringe will sometimes be of some value as a method of collecting sperm, although the amount obtained will be very small.

Another method is to force some of the fluid out of the seminal vesicles and through the urethra by means of massaging the prostate gland.

Moral Aspect: There is no moral objection to either aspiration by needle or prostate massage because neither of these methods includes any exercise of the generative faculty as such.

Some authors express the liceity of these two methods as only probable,[262] but it is difficult to see any valid argument contrary to it.

Morally the removal of sperm for examination by aspiration or prostate massage does not differ from the removal of a blood specimen from the body for a blood count.

Perforated Condom to Collect Sperm: Intercourse between husband and wife, with the husband using a condom which has been perforated in such a way that some of the semen is deposited in his wife's vagina, while some remains in the condom to be collected later for examination, is a method whereby a reasonable specimen of seminal fluid can be obtained.

Moral Aspect: This unique and admittedly very clinical approach to the marital act has been employed satisfactorily by some physicians and has likewise been defended reasonably by some moralists. Father J. McCarthy, of Maynooth College in Ireland, wrote as follows:

> In the normal ejaculate there is a vast number of spermatozoa—one of which suffices for fecundation. Consequently, the use in intercourse of a condom which is sufficiently perforated to allow the deposition of a considerable portion of the ejaculate in the vagina of the woman cannot be said to make the act inept for generation. In other words, in this hypothesis of sufficient perforation, intercourse with a punctured condom is an 'act of itself suitable for the generation of offspring.' The intercourse is substantially undistorted and natural. The procreation of offspring is not artificially prevented. It does not follow, of course, that intercourse with a perforated condom is always lawful. The procedure does involve some degree of interference with the natural act and, perhaps, some slight lessening of the chances of subsequent fecundation. All this would clearly be somehow unlawful if there is no justifying cause. If the seminal specimens obtained by using a punctured condom are really useful for sterility tests and may thus be helpful toward curing sterile conditions—then there is present, we think, a sufficiently grave cause to justify the method.[263]

In the above quotation Father McCarthy might have been somewhat underestimating the degree to which fertility potential is liable to be lessened by considerable lessening of the amount of sperm deposited in the vagina in an individual act of intercourse. This, however, does not necessarily destroy the validity of his argument, particularly since studies seem to indicate that the concentration of the ejaculate is of far more importance than the amount in the fertility potential of an act of intercourse.[264]

We have already seen that Father Clifford links the use of a punctured condom as a proposed solution for impotence in some cases of hypospadias to the present question, and approves of the use of the perforated condom in such circumstances.

The real nub of the moral question here would seem to be whether or not intercourse with a sufficiently perforated condom is, of itself, an act suitable for the generation of offspring. If it is, then it is difficult to see how such an act, done not with contraceptive intent, but with contra-sterility intent, is totally and substantially vitiated by a partial loss of sperm.

Therefore, we would hold that sperm collection by means of intercourse between husband and wife, with a condom so perforated as to allow sufficient sperm to be deposited in the vagina to permit conception, is certainly permitted in practice.

Extraction of Sperm from the Vagina: Another method of obtaining sperm specimen for examination is to have a married couple perform marital intercourse and then permit the doctor to collect some of the sperm from the woman's vagina by means of a syringe.

Moral Aspect: It would seem that the same arguments brought forth in defense of the use of the perforated condom demonstrate, with even greater force, the liceity of this procedure. It does not seem that the removal of some sperm immediately or very soon after coitus can be said to negative the marriage act or to substantially impair its aptitude for the generation of offspring, particularly in view of the fact that sperm has been found in the uterus within three minutes after intercourse.[265]

Therefore, recognizing a difference of opinion in this matter among the moralists, we can say that it is solidly probable in theory and certain in practice that this method of sperm collection is permitted.

Interruption of Intercourse after Partial Insemination: Some physicians have suggested a sort of interrupted ejaculate as a possible method for collecting sperm. This technique would consist in having a husband and wife begin the marital act and continue until part of the ejaculate has been deposited in the vagina. Whereupon the husband would withdraw and deposit the remainder of the ejaculate in a sterile receptacle, for future examination.

Moral Aspect: The argument advanced to defend the morality of this procedure is based on the premise that such an act does leave conception possible, and that therefore the act remains substantially one which is, of itself, suitable for the generation of offspring.

This represents an approach to the moral problem along a proper line of reasoning. However, it overlooks the significance of the interruption of the act itself. And because this method involves a violent and unnatural deordination of the very act of intercourse we cannot grant any moral probability in its favor.

Moreover, there are morally acceptable methods of obtaining sperm which involve much less a deordination of the marital act, and it must be remembered that the medically acceptable method which least alters the act of intercourse itself would necessarily be the method of moral choice.

The Cervical Spoon: At about the turn of the century, Dr. Joseph B. Doyle, Director of the Sterility Clinic at Saint Elizabeth's Hospital in Boston and Assistant in Obstetrics at Tufts Medical College, reported on the use of the cervical spoon for collecting sperm. His report, in part, is as follows:

> A concave lucite spoon has been devised to provide an innocuous inner lining of the posterior fornix and vaginal wall. It is inserted in the vaginal canal, its shaft gently depressed by flexion of the index finger against the relaxed perineum and posterior vaginal wall as the patient gently bears down. The cervix can be digitally felt as it dips into the spoon . . . Before coitus, the husband places the spoon (which has first been washed in hot tap water and allowed to dry) beneath the cervix. Intromission from above is readily attained . . .
>
> "[after coitus] the wife remains supine for at least an hour. Then the spoon is withdrawn by the husband as the wife gently bears down to relax the perineum. The contents of the 'seminal spoon pool,' liquified ejaculate plus minimal cervical mucus and a trace of vaginal secretion, are deposited in a clean boiled glass jar for study of viscosity, sperm count, morphology, and viability . . . Spoon semen samples collected after the spoon was left one to five hours in the vagina

show fifty to eighty per cent of the sperm active. Fresh specimens withdrawn within thirty minutes and left standing in the spoon within a large stoppered jar for five hours at room temperature show little change in motility, indicating that the lucite spoon is not deleterious to the sperm."[266]

Moral Aspect: Although this method never gained wide clinical acceptance, a brief moral evaluation of it serves to illustrate the principles involved. At the time of ordinary coitus direct insemination of the cervix is very unlikely. Actually most of the ejaculate collects in a pool at the base of the cervix. As the cervical mucus drips down to make contact with this pool, the sperm that have survived the acid vaginal secretions can make their way through the ejaculate secretions to the cervical mucus and through the os cervicis.

The lucite spoon serves to protect the sperm from the vaginal acids, and collect it at the bottom of the cervix, and thus renders the marriage act itself more, rather than less, likely to result in conception.

Therefore, granted an interval of time between coitus and the removal of the spoon sufficient to permit sperm to pass the os cervicis in a supply adequate to effect possible generation, we see no possibility of any reasonable objection to this method of sperm collection.

An Important Notation: Some of the methods of sperm collection described above have, at times, met an attitude of clinical disdain on the part of some physicians. Let it be remembered that it has been physicians who have submitted these methods to theologians for moral evaluation.

Artificial Insemination

The general term of "artificial insemination" is used to include any process outside the purely natural act of intercourse which might be employed to bring about the fecundation of an ovum.

The practice of artificial insemination has been known to animal husbandry for many centuries. The commonly accepted first case among humans was reported only at the end of the

eighteenth century (1799) when the wife of an English mer-
chant was successfully inseminated with her husband's sperm
under the direction of one John Hunter. Others claim Robert
Dickinson was the pioneer in human artificial insemination in
1890, and there are those who identify the practice among the
Jews as early as the second century.[267]

Although the current medical literature reflects a reluctance
on the part of many physicians to engage themselves in the
various legal, moral and genetic complications of artificial insemination, there is also evidence that it is not extremely difficult to find established doctors who are willing to assist in the
process.

In modern clinical practice the source of sperm for artificial
insemination has most frequently been the anonymous donor,
although sometimes the oligospermatic husband's ejaculate is
reinforced with a mixture of donor sperm.

Although frozen sperm has been used in animal husbandry
for many years, very little had been done with such techniques
in the field of human reproduction until fairly recently. Perloff,
Steinberger and Sherman reported successful pregnancies with
spermatozoa which had been stored in liquid nitrogen for almost
six months, and subsequently up to ten months. Fernandez-Cano,
Menkin, Garcia and Rock reported successful pregnancies with
spermatozoa which had been stored at minus 70 degrees C., with
glycol as a protective agent.

Moral Aspects: The moral aspects of artificial insemination
presented here are derived from the teaching of the Catholic
Church on the subject. This teaching is mainly embodied in the
papal allocution of Pius XII to the Fourth International Congress
of Catholic Doctors, given at Castel Gandolfo, September 29,
1949.[268]

Before reviewing these moral aspects in detail, it is necessary
to determine a concise terminology in this matter. The very real
difference between "artificial insemination" and "artificial aids
to fecundation," in a moral context, must be clearly understood.

Artificial Insemination: By artificial insemination we mean
any process whereby the male spermatozoa is brought into juxta-

position with the female ovum by any means apart from and wholly distinct from the natural act of marital intercourse. All such means will be seen to be contrary to the papal teaching.

Artificial Aids to Fecundation: By artificial aids to fecundation we mean the various methods of assisting the natural act of marital intercourse to achieve the impregnation of the female ovum. It will be seen that such artificial aids have not received any wholesale condemnation.

The following quotations from the papal allocution present the teaching of Pius XII on the various aspects of the problem.

Artificial insemination outside of marriage: The evident moral aberration involved in the concept of artificial insemination outside of marriage was described as follows by Pius XII:

> Artificial fecundation outside of marriage must be purely and simply condemned as immoral . . . Such indeed is the natural and the divine positive law, that the procreation of a new life can come only as the fruit of marriage. Marriage alone safeguards the dignity of the parents (especially, in the present case, of the wife), it alone safeguards their personal welfare . . . Of itself, marriage alone provides for the welfare and education of the child.

Artificial insemination within marriage with the active element of a third party: This concept is no less a travesty of the sacredness of marriage, and is likewise rejected by the papal teaching:

> Artificial fecundation within marriage, but produced by the active element of a third party is equally immoral and as such deserves unqualified condemnation . . . The parents alone have a reciprocal right over each other's body to engender a new life, and this right is exclusive, perpetual, and inalienable. And this is as it should be, in consideration also of the child. Nature imposes upon the one who gives life to a little being, in virtue of this bond between them, the task of conservation and education. But between the legitimate husband and that child, which, with his consent, is the fruit of the active element of a third party, there exists no bond of origin, no moral and juridical bond of conjugal procreation.

Legal Aspects of Donor Artificial Insemination: In the

United States some courts have viewed donor artificial insemination as adultery, and grounds for divorce, although there is some question as to how most states could interpret donor insemination as adultery, since so many of them explicitly include carnal copula in their definition of that crime. Moreover, in a few cases donor insemination children have been declared illegitimate by the courts. This immediately confuses the question of inheritance and support, which is further complicated by the consideration of how these questions would be answered if the identity of the donor were to be established.

To date the courts have had little or nothing to say on the legal position of the doctor in cases of donor insemination. But where the insemination is done without the knowledge of one or other of the parties concerned, one can easily see possible action against the physician for damages, assault or battery, or even a medical misdemeanor. Moreover, in order to protect the secret of donor insemination, the physician is quite likely to be maneuvered into making a false entry on the birth certificate, for which he would be held legally accountable.

Artificial insemination within marriage with the active element of the proper spouse: Before the publication of the papal allocution of Pope Pius XII, a number of moralists held, as at least probable, that strictly artificial insemination between husband and wife could be permitted provided the husband's sperm was obtained in some legitimate way.

This doctrine, however, is no longer tenable. Pius XII pointed out that such a pregnancy would not render valid a marriage between persons unable to contract marriage because of the impediment of impotence and at the same time he condemned outright all strictly artificial insemination:

Although we cannot 'a priori' exclude new methods solely because of their novelty, nevertheless in what concerns artificial fecundation there is not merely room for extreme caution, but it must absolutely be avoided . . . Only the procreation of a new life according to the will and plan of the Creator carries with it the realization of the ends that are sought, and it does so with a remarkable degree of perfection. Such procreation is, at the same time, in conformity with the corporal and spiritual nature and the dignity of the spouses, and with the normal and felicitous development of the child.

In the supposition that the insemination would be with the husband's sperm, which was collected in a morally accepted manner, the moral evil of artificial insemination arises from a deordination in the manner of human generation.

We might recall here that the two most significant and important events in the history of the human race were its creation and its redemption. Both of these acts were performed by God alone. But God, seeing man's need of continued creation and constant redemption, has, in His merciful condescension, willed to continue these acts, and to renew them, with man's cooperation. They have both been sanctified in the sacramental form, and here one can discern a beautiful analogy between matrimony and holy orders.

Without extending the analogy beyond its proper proportions, we can understand the impact, within the moral order, of the sacredness of the renewal of God's redemptive act in the Sacrifice of the Mass and of God's creative act in the generation of a child, and appreciate the moral propriety of the *modus agendi* in each instance.

And a source no less authoritative than the papal teaching itself has pointed out that in this awesome act of generation, so reflective of the divine power and beauty and so expressive of all that is God-like in human nature, any substantial deviation from the natural and beautifully intimate conjugal union is to be condemned as inconsonant with the sanctity of that sublime act wherein God and man, in concausality, renew God's creative act.

Human Fecundation in vitro : Experimentation designed to unite the human sperm and ovum *in vitro*, whatever hope it may offer to advance genetic knowledge, must be condemned as immoral.

Aside from the extreme moral impropriety of laboratory fecundation, in the light of the preceding evaluation of artificial insemination, the fertilized human ovum must be treated as an inviolable human life from the moment of conception. In this latter concept, Father Gerald Kelly, S.J., and Father John Ford, S.J., recognized the moral evil of *in vitro* fecundation as comparable to that of abortion, merely pushing the expulsion of the non-viable fetus back to the very beginning of its embryonic life,[269] since the products of such conception cannot long survive. We might also point out that, in view of the probability of the immediate hominization, this type of experimentation is in direct conflict with that accepted norm of the entire medical profession which condemns any experiment "which is undertaken when there is real reason to believe that death or serious injury will result."

Finally, in his allocution to the Second World Congress on Fertility and Sterility (May 19, 1956) Pope Pius XII stated:

"On the subject of the experiments in artificial human fecundation *in vitro*, let it suffice for us to observe that they must be rejected as immoral and absolutely illicit."[270]

Even aside from the concise papal evaluation of artificial fecundation, whether *in vivo* or *in vitro*, this type of wanton experimentation with human life at its very point of origin is so divorced from even a fundamental reverence for humanity and society, and so expressive of the materialistic mind, as to justly merit Father Joseph Donovan's description: "Test-tube conception and test-tube murder are the last work of a dying civilization."[271]

Dr. Schellen draws a vivid picture, throughout his book, of the social destructiveness and moral dangers of artificial insemination in all its forms,[272] and Father Gerald Kelly, S.J., commenting on the reported desirable moral and intellectual character of the apt donor, justly questioned the morality and intellectuality of any man who would "calmly enter a doctor's office or laboratory and ejaculate semen into a glass jar for a sum of money." Father Kelly further commented:

... and whose realization of the responsibilities of parenthood (would be) so slight that he would be willing to father a child, or many children, whom he would never see

and towards whom he would have no duty—and this, moreover, through a woman he does not even know . . . The donor,
whatever be his other qualifications, can hardly be either
psychologically or morally normal.[273]

Artificial Aids to Fecundation: There is the distinction, no
less evident to the physician than it is important to the theologian, between artificial insemination and artificial aids to the
natural act of fecundation. Pope Pius XII recognized this distinction in his address to the Fourth International Congress of
Catholic Doctors in the following significant statement:

> By speaking this way, (i.e., that artificial insemination is
> to be entirely rejected), we do not necessarily forbid the use
> of artificial means whose sole purpose is either to facilitate
> the natural act or to assist the natural act, placed normally,
> in attaining its purpose.

Under this heading of artificial aids to natural fecundation
we would immediately classify the use of the perforated condom
to correct hypospadias, the lucite spoon used as an aid to sperm
migration, and the collection of sperm in a syringe immediately
after marital intercourse in order to propel it toward the cervix.

An intriguing possibility presents itself in cases of sterility
due to the husband's oligospermia. It is possible to collect amounts
of the husband's ejaculate, by morally acceptable methods, in
proper acts of intercourse. These amounts can be conserved and
spun down, leaving a residue containing a heavy concentration
of viable spermatozoa. There are several ways whereby this
concentrated deposit of active sperm could be placed within the
generative tract of the wife, immediately before a natural marital
act, in order to mix with and fortify the husband's ejaculate.

Although this type of procedure would undoubtedly give rise
to some difference of opinion among theologians, we believe
that, in view of the explicit papal distinction regarding "artificial
means whose sole purpose is either to facilitate the natural act or
to assist the natural act, placed normally, in attaining its purpose,"
it could be permitted in practice.

Rebound Therapy: Temporary suppression of spermatogenesis in the male has offered some promise as a therapy to remedy oligospermia in cases of male infertility. Administration of testosterone to the male results in a sharp limitation of spermatogenesis and if the hormone treatment is continued complete azoospermia may result in about twelve weeks. Then, when testosterone is discontinued, as the spermatogenesis reactivates after two or three months a "rebound phenomenon" sometimes occurs and the production of spermatozoa is increased over its previous level.[274]

Moral Comment: At first glance rebound testosterone therapy for oligospermia might seem to present a moral problem, since the spermatogenic function is directly suppressed and this indeed may seem to be a direct, though temporary, pharmacuological sterilization.

The rebound therapy, however, is used only in cases where the patient is already essentially sterile, due to his oligospermic condition.

The further temporary suppression of a spermatogenic function which is already presumed enfeebled below the level of fertility, as a means to achieve future fertility, cannot be classified as an immoral mutilation. It is scarcely an attack on the functional efficiency of the generative system since this generative system has no functional efficiency.

The rebound therapy simply does not contain that deordination of nature which specifies a direct sterilization within the generative system as immoral. Hence it does not fall within the ambit of the Church's condemnation of direct sterilization and, on the contrary, is actually a morally praiseworthy procedure in the interest of future functional integrity.

Breast Feeding

From time to time the question is asked: whether or not a mother has a moral obligation to suckle her newborn child, if she can do so. The moral theologians have not written extensively on the question and there is, in the medical literature, considerable disparity of opinion as to the advantages of breast feeding. The standard obstetric texts that deal with the subject strongly favor breast feeding. Note the two following examples:

Eastman: The ideal food for the newborn child is the milk of its mother, and, unless lactation is contraindicated by some physical defect, it is the physician's duty to urge every woman at least to attempt to suckle her child . . . The act itself also exerts a beneficial influence upon the involution of the uterus since it is well known that the repeated irritation of the nipples results in reflex stimulation of the uterus.[275]

Cunningham: The importance of breast-feeding is universally recognized and cannot be overestimated. In the absence of a definite contraindication, the doctor should always advise and encourage it, even where the patient, the nurse and the relations are opposed to it. Not only the welfare but, in some cases, the life of the child may depend on it.[276]

In the journals, however, one finds articles which stress the value of breast feeding for the health and immunity of the infant and other articles which attempt to prove that such claims have been very much overemphasized and that, in general, the bottle-fed baby does about as well as the breast-fed baby.

No moral question arises in those cases where one of the various medical contraindications to breast feeding is identified. These include such things as infant allergy to the mother's milk, failure of sufficient caloric content, fissured nipples, mastitis, or malignancy, acute maternal illness, pregnancy, excessive pain, maternal tuberculosis and some doubtful contraindications such as Rh factor incompatibility.

The moral question is: what obligation does a mother have to suckle her child when there is no medical contraindication to this and she can do it with relatively little inconvenience?

In evaluating this question one must remember that before the days of perfected baby formula and at a time when whole milk was not sterilized and processed as it is today, breast feeding was, in many cases, the only truly safe nutrition for a newborn. This is no longer true in most areas of the United States.

Moreover a natural reluctance on the part of the mother to suckle the infant is likely to affect the actual organic supply and delivery of nutrition and thus interfere with the process to the detriment of the child.

Nor is there agreement among the medical specialists that breast-feeding offers any notable psychic advantages for the infant over proper and affectionate bottle-feeding.

Thus we believe that aside from some special need, medical, pediatric and psychiatric opinions on the advantages to the newborn of breast feeding over bottle feeding are not sufficiently established to impose any obligation on the mother to suckle her infant. At the same time, however, there is sufficient indication of advantages of breast feeding that the physician might do well to encourage the practice whenever he deems it feasible.

Masturbation

The accepted medical definition of masturbation identifies the act with "self-pollution" or the production of sexual orgasm by some mechanical friction distinct from an act of intercourse.

The theological evaluation, in Catholic teaching, adds the dimension that masturbation is a serious distortion of the basic beauty and dignity of human sexuality, as well as a totally self-referenced turning inward of this most fundamentally communicative aspect of human love. This moral disorder often escapes comprehension in our contemporary atmosphere of ethical materialism, in which a "victimless crime" is not considered to be criminal or wrong (even if the victim is one's self).

The Catholic Church teaches that, objectively, masturbation is a sin. The fact that many physicians reject this notion again illustrates how our popular morality has become more sociological than theological. Although "social order" is a very important criterion of morality, when "social order" displaces "God's law" in ethical orientation, the basic dignity of the human person suffers.

The thoughtful man, who regards human nature in its totality and in its diversified relationships, should have no difficulty recognizing the reproductive faculty as oriented toward the generation and education of offspring in the context of the family; and this from every biological, psychological, and sociological consideration. He can further readily appreciate why deviations in so important a matter would be seriously sinful. These same truths of the natural law are nuanced in divine revelation.[277]

The moralist adds the notion of "directly voluntary" to the medical definition of masturbation and so distinguishes it from the natural discharge of sexual tension which may occur during sleep and from accidentally or unintentionally induced episodes during waking hours. Even here, however, it must be pointed out that to positively accept or seek the resultant venereal sensation actually contributes to and furthers the exercise of the generative faculty and thus becomes integrated with the moral turpitude of contributing to and promoting continuance of the masturbatory act.

It should be clearly understood that the malice of masturbation consists primarily in the deliberate exercise of the generative faculty outside of a proper marriage act and not precisely in the experiencing of venereal pleasure, except insofar as consent to such is automatically contributory to the increased intensity of the act itself. Thus even if a physician were to induce pollution in a semi-conscious patient (to obtain a sperm sample, or for any other reason) with no venereal pleasure experienced by the patient, the objective malice of the act of masturbation would remain unchanged and the moral guilt would be incurred by the physician, as well as by the patient if he had previously agreed to the procedure.

The good physician, charged with the over-all welfare of the sick, should render whatever encouragement and assistance he can to help a patient who is a victim of this habit overcome his problem. At the same time the physician should be aware of the psychopathologic overtones of the masturbatory mind. The element of habit superimposed upon personality disorientation can certainly compromise the voluntariety of the practice and thus lessen the subjective culpability.

Moreover the physician himself must be careful to keep his own attitude in this matter in accord with proper moral concepts. The current medical literature is not without examples of a completely materialistic view which identifies this moral disorder simply as a "taboo," or as a normal phenomenon which has become encrusted with "religious scruples." Levine and Bell, for example, write as follows about masturbation. Without agreeing with their evaluation of the subject, one might note that even they do not completely exclude the overtones of abnormality.

An examination of the literature reveals that until very recently this activity was considered as 'very bad' and one to be prohibited at all costs . . . Again we find our cultural attitudes erecting prohibitions. Just as feces are considered dirty and poisonous, as mentioned in our previous paper, so masturbation is considered sinful. To complicate matters even further, various religious sects prohibit masturbation . . . Although masturbatory activity in childhood may be considered as entirely normal, and in adolescence as a normal outlet for suppressed heterosexual urges, excessive masturbation cannot be considered normal at any age level. . . .[278]

A certain masturbatory phase has been identified in small children as occurring around the age of 4 to 6 years, and then quiescing until the pre-adolescent period.

Although the pediatric masturbator is not guilty of formal sin, the act of masturbation does remain an objective deorientation of the natural law. The moral problem arises with the consideration of the responsibility on the part of the competent adults, such as parents, physicians, etc.

In view of the medical consideration of possible psychic trauma in the child which may become manifest later and may be due either to a wrong method of correcting the infantile situation, or not correcting it at all, the following moral observations are in order:

1. An objective violation of the natural law may sometimes be permitted for a very serious reason, is never to be encouraged, and is normally to be corrected. This norm is particularly applicable in those instances where, due to immaturity or amentia, there is no formal guilt.
2. Thus in certain isolated instances of individual masturbatory acts of an infant or a severe psychotic, there might

be proportionate medical indications to passively permit the action.

3. Even in these cases the action can never be initiated or encouraged, even as a therapeutic measure.

Vaginal Tampons and Menstrual Hygiene

The popular use of vaginal tampons for menstrual hygiene did not begin until the mid-1930's, and it is interesting to note that the substitution of the vaginal tampon for the conventional external pad very quickly became a moral issue in Great Britain. Some British theologians, undoubtedly basing their judgments on the views of some contemporary medical opinions, condemned the use of tampons as physically harmful and morally dangerous.[279] These same views have been shared by not a few American gynecologists.[280] The harmful physical effects referred to included possible trauma to the hymen and/or the vaginal mucosa, damming of menstrual flow, and introduction of infectious organisms into the vagina. The moral danger was seen as erotic stimulation by the necessary manipulations for inserting and removing the tampon and possible phallic symbolism.

On the other hand there are those who felt that these difficulties had been much overemphasized. Beginning in 1939, Dr. Madeline Thornton of the University of Wisconsin School of Medicine, did an extensive study of one hundred and ten women using vaginal tampons over a period of from one to two years. The subjects were questioned and examined every two months and the conclusions of this study were that there was no evidence of tampon irritation of the cervix or vagina, or of obstruction to menstrual flow, or any acquired trichonomas or yeast infections.[281]

Moral Aspects: As to the question of the morality of the use of vaginal tampons during menstruation in relation to any unnecessary risk to health or physical well-being, the matter must be left entirely to the good judgment of the individual physician and the individual patient. There is certainly no sufficiency of scientific evidence today that would warrant the moralist's general condemnation of the use of vaginal tampons as injurious to health.

The question of erotic stimulation by insertion of the tampon was discussed in the literature under two aspects: stimulation by local irritation of sensory nerve endings and the possibility of some psychic stimulation by phallic suggestion.[282]

Regarding local stimulation, Dr. Robert Dickinson pointed out, in the *Journal of the American Medical Association*, that tampons are much less likely to give rise to erotic feelings than are sanitary pads. They are placed in an area in the vagina where nerve endings are so few that it is possible to perform minor surgery in this area without anesthesia.[283]

The question of psychic stimulation by phallic suggestion is not very practical. Physicians consulted on this point do not feel there is much danger of such erotic stimulation. If it is present, it is likely to be due to the subjective dispositions of the user, a symptom calling for psychiatric consultation, or at least spiritual direction.

Vaginal Douche after Marital Intercourse: Sometimes questions are asked regarding the use of a vaginal douche after marital intercourse for reasons of cleanliness, general hygiene, or comfort, or with some specific medical indication, and apart from any contraceptive intention.

A number of the standard moralists have contraindicated a douche employed for reasons of cleanliness or comfort up to from three to four to ten or twelve hours after copula, and they would permit such a douche for serious medical reasons not before one hour after copula. This opinion is clearly summarized in Father Charles McFadden's *Medical Ethics*:

> If the purpose of the douche is cleanliness, health, or other reasonable good, no moral objection is made to the use of a douche after three or four hours have elapsed since marital intercourse, for during that time the process of nature would normally have had its effect.
>
> In serious and extraordinary cases, where reasons of health demand it, the use of a douche one hour after marital intercourse may be permitted.[284]

In view of the time element involved in normal sperm migration, it would appear that this opinion is too strict. In advising a patient in this matter one could certainly follow the older and more realistic opinion of Vermeersch and permit vaginal douche for reasons of health, cleanliness, or comfort after a reasonable interval has elapsed from the time of intercourse.

Vermeersch: "When done for some other purpose (i.e., other than as a contraceptive measure) a vaginal douche now seems to be permitted one hour after intercourse, since then it does not impede conception. . .

". . . After a half hour or an hour enough nemaspermata has been received into the uterus to fulfill the morally expected hope of fecundation. . . ."[285]

Moreover if, for some very serious medical reason, a physician would judge it necessary to prescribe a vaginal douche earlier, or even immediately after intercourse, this could be done under the principle of double effect. Obviously the "serious reason" cannot be of a contraceptive nature.

Vaginal Douche after Rape: In the event that a woman, herself unwilling, has suffered violent and unjust attack, she may use a vaginal douche as soon as possible, with the intention of ridding herself of the sperm which has been unjustly deposited in her vagina.

The invading sperm under these circumstances is merely the continuation of an unjust aggression, and can be treated accordingly. Unlike her husband's seed, this sperm is unjustly present within her body. The aggressor had no right to place it there and she has no obligation to receive or retain it.

Note that we are dealing here only with a vaginal douche to exclude invading spermatozoa. We have already seen, earlier in this chapter, that the use of the so-called "morning after pill" or dilation and curretage to insure the subsequent destruction of a possible conceptus (embryo) carries with it the moral malice of abortion.

CHAPTER SEVEN

PROFESSIONAL SECRECY

One of the most sacred obligations of the physician is his duty to observe professional secrecy, that is, to have a profound respect for the confidences entrusted to him by his patients. Two of the most fundamental and significant writings in the history of Medical Ethics have been the Hippocratic collection and the Code of Medical Ethics which Dr. Thomas Percival brought forth out of the administrative turmoil of the Manchester Infirmary, in England, at the close of the eighteenth century. The concept of professional secrecy is prominent in each of these sources.

The Hippocratic collection clearly reflects how sacred and serious the obligation of secrecy has been held from the dawn of medical history. This is expressed strongly and succinctly in the words of the traditional oath: ". . . whatever I shall see or hear in the course of my profession, as well as outside my profession in my intercourse with men, if it be what should not be published abroad, I will never divulge, holding such things to be holy secrets. . ."

Percival's observations on professional secrecy were capsulated in the following sentences: "Secrecy and delicacy, when required by peculiar circumstances, should be strictly observed. And the familiar and confidential intercourse, to which the faculty are admitted in their professional visits, should be used with discretion and with the most scrupulous regard to fidelity and honor."[286]

Half a century later, when the American Medical Association held its first formal meeting in Philadelphia (May 1847) and adopted its original Code of Ethics, the delegates simply took the above quotation from Percival and added the following:

The obligation of secrecy extends beyond the period of professional services; none of the privacies of personal or domestic life, no infirmity of disposition or flaw of character observed during professional attendance, should ever be divulged by him (the physician) except when he is imperatively required to do so. The force and necessity of this obligation are indeed so great, that professional men have, under certain circumstances, been protected in their observance of secrecy by courts of justice.[287]

As the AMA Code of Ethics was revised and rearranged in 1903, 1912, 1947, and 1955, the section on professional secrecy remained essentially intact. And when, in 1957, the House of Delegates adopted a radically new form of expression of the "Principles of Ethics," designed to eliminate various dicta of mere etiquette which were scattered among the ethical directives, section nine became a summary of all that had previously been held regarding professional secrecy, and reads as follows: "A physician may not reveal the confidences entrusted to him in the course of medical attendance, or the deficiencies he may observe in the character of patients, unless he is required to do so by law or unless it becomes necessary to protect the welfare of the individual or of the community."[288]

Theologians commonly distinguish various kinds of secrets and obligations arising from them. Before going into the details of the natural secret, the promised secret, and the committed secret, as well as the professional secret, it will be advisable to consider the natural law basis for the obligations of secrecy in general.

Obligation of Secrecy Based on Natural Law: Considering that the natural law is merely the divine Will of the Creator as promulgated by the human conscience, and that we learn a great deal about the Will of the Creator by a consideration of the things that are created and the purpose for which they are created, we can discover the foundations to the rights and obligations of secrecy by an inspection of man, considered both as an individual and as a member of society.

Considering man as an individual, we find that the Author of nature has indicated the right to secrecy merely by providing the higher faculties of man with a natural inviolability which, under normal circumstances and apart from unjust means, no other human being is physically able to penetrate. God alone is the reader of hearts, as we read in the seventh psalm; or in the words of God to Samuel: "for man seeth the things that appear, but the Lord beholdeth the heart." (2 K 16:7)

Among the earlier writers, DeLugo pointed out that the inviolability of the secret from this aspect does not depend on any consideration of circumstances or social welfare, but is due to the very nature of man.[289]

Moreover, it is obvious that those things which are the product of man's own labor, with his own tools, in his own goods or in the common possessions of men, are his own.

Thus the knowledge and the thoughts which a man has, and which pertain only to himself, are his own. The fact that he has a right to his own thoughts and ideas is recognized as the basis of copyright and patent law.

Hence we see that the subject matter of the right is knowledge, ideas, or thoughts; and the scope of the right is possession, use, or disposal according to the will of the owner, and with due consideration for the rights of others.

Man is necessarily and by nature a social being. Thus we see the necessity of secrecy from the viewpoint of man as a member of society. For the proper development of his natural powers and the harmonious fulfillment of his natural drives, man has to live in society with other men.

It is in this regard that Thomas Aquinas points out the following:

> One man naturally owes to another that without which human society cannot be preserved . . . men cannot live together unless they are truthful with one another . . . Truthfulness stands in the mean between too much and too little.[290]

Vermeersch developed the same idea in these words:

> Since both extremes must be avoided as sinful, namely, failure to tell the truth when it ought to be told and indiscreet revealing of the truth, the means of virtue is to be followed. This is obtained by observing the law of sincerity,

which induces discreet manifestation of the truth; and by the law of secrecy, which prohibits indiscreet manifestation of the truth.[291]

DeLugo brought out another aspect of the necessity of proper secrecy for the public peace and prosperity, which is required in order that men might live together in society:

Thus we cannot properly inquire about the crimes and secret defects of our neighbor, or broadcast them. For this is very destructive of the public peace and tranquility. Moreover, that these crimes remain occult and be buried in ignorance and oblivion helps toward avoiding crime and gently correcting faults. Because the conserving of one's good name is a great control and motive for good living, and when that control has been removed and a man's reputation is once lost, human frailty rushes easily and precipitously into desperation, since the hope of preserving a good reputation among men is gone.[292]

Robert Regan, closer to our own time and culture, but writing along the same lines observed the following precisely with regard to the professional secret and the common good:

To cut men off from the support of their fellow men would tend to disorganize and disrupt society; whereas a properly functioning social life, as previously pointed out, is demanded by man's very nature. In certain difficulties men are forced to turn for assistance to others better qualified than themselves. Assurance that they will not be betrayed, and thus find their sorry condition made worse, is a necessary condition for this recourse. For if the needy and unfortunate are persuaded that in their misfortunes they cannot look to others for assistance without the danger of betrayal which will bring down upon them even greater evils, such as loss of fortune, loss of reputation and honor, great embarrassment, loss of liberty, and even loss of life itself, they will prefer to keep their troubles to themselves. Thus frustration would most certainly engender hopelessness, despondency, and despair, with the fruits of such states of mind and soul, such as recklessness and dereliction of duty. The evils that would befall society if such conditions existed could be enormous.[293]

Various Kinds of Secrets: Because the proper concept of the professional secret is not only closely allied to, but also intertwined with, the other types of secrets, a brief explanation of all of these is in order.

The Purely Natural Secret: The purely natural secret can be described as a secret whose obligation arises from the nature of the matter, without a contract; because, for example, the thing which someone knows by chance cannot be manifested without someone else being reasonably unwilling.

The obligation of the purely natural secret would be in charity if the only effect of revealing the secret would be the reasonable displeasure of the one whom it concerns. This obligation would be light or serious according to the degree of reasonable displeasure which would be caused to the one concerned if he knew that his secret were revealed.

If, however, in addition to the displeasure, the revelation would bring damage to reputation or material loss to the one concerned, the purely natural secret would oblige also in justice; and the obligation would be light or grave according to the loss liable to be incurred.

The Promised Secret: The promised secret is one whose obligation arises from a promise not to divulge certain information, the promise being made by one who already is in possession of the information in question.

Since the promise is made, either spontaneously or upon request, only after the secret is already known to the one promising, it is obvious that the obligation is based on the virtue of fidelity only, and therefore obliges only in so far as the person making the promise intended to oblige himself, unless the nature of the matter makes the promised secret also a natural secret.

The Committed Secret: The committed secret is one whose obligation arises from a contract made before the secret knowledge is imparted, and as a condition under which it is imparted. The "quid pro quo" which is required in any contract comes down to this: that the possessor of the secret says, in effect: "I will give you this knowledge of mine if you will give me the assurance of its absolute security." The wills of the contracting parties meet in one and the same object, namely, the secret knowledge.

Thus it is clear that the obligation of the committed secret arises from an onerous contract, and binds in justice. If the matter of the secret is of sufficient moment, the obligation is considered to be a very serious one.

There are, however, circumstances in which the committed secret may be revealed, as for example: to protect the common good, or when its revelation is required to avert harm which is unjustly being brought against an innocent third party by the one who committed the secret. The innocent party has a right to be defended against an unjust wrong.

Obviously the committed secret can also be a natural secret.

The Professional Secret: The professional secret is a committed secret, binding in justice, wherein the contract of secrecy is not explicitly put into words, but is implicit by reason of the professional position of the one who receives the secret knowledge.

There is no doubt regarding the necessity of the medical profession for the common good, or the fact that people sometimes have to reveal their secrets to doctors, and that these secrets have to be kept inviolate in order that the medical profession may properly fulfill its function and that people may have free and easy access to doctors.

Therefore, when a doctor enters the practice of medicine he makes an implicit contract with all who come to him in his professional capacity: that whatever secrets they impart to him in the professional doctor-patient relationship will be kept inviolate, and will be used only in so far as necessary to achieve the purpose for which the patient entered into this relationship.

Basic Principle I: The professional person is obliged to keep the secrets of his clients as long as the client retains the right to the secret.

It will be recalled that the first source of this obligation is founded in the concept of the natural secret, based on the individual's natural right, as an individual, and irrespective of the added obligation of professional secrecy, which is more specifically founded on the concept of the common good.

The secret, as a natural secret, is the property of the patient, and when the patient makes his secret known to the doctor he does not renounce his title to that property. Because of the implicit contract of the professional relationship, he merely assigns a limited use of that property to the professional person; namely, that use and only that use which the professional person has to make of the secret knowledge in order that he may accomplish the purpose for which the patient entered into the professional relationship with him.

It is this strict limitation on the professional use of the knowledge which adds the formal note of "professional secret" to the "natural secret." And this added obligation of the "professional secret" is based on the fact that it is extremely necessary for the common good that people have free and easy access to the assistance of the profession, without fear of their secrets being betrayed.

This dual aspect of "professional" and "natural" secrecy is of considerable importance. In an individual case, even though the doctor may realize that some information which he has concerning a patient does not come under the heading of professional secrecy, he may still find himself obliged to observe natural secrecy.

It has been previously mentioned that there are circumstances which permit, or even require, the revelation of the professional secret. The second and third basic principles deal with these circumstances.

Basic Principle II: Private property, including a secret, becomes common in common necessity.

Since the obligation of professional secrecy comes about because the observance of professional secrecy is a necessary means to preserve the common good and the right order of society, if a set of conditions and circumstances should be found in which the observance of professional secrecy would, in particular cases, be more harmful than helpful for the common good, then the obligation of secrecy would cease and the obligation to reveal the secret would take its place.

In such a case the individual's right to natural secrecy would vanish because private property becomes common in common necessity.

Moreover, the added communal right to professional secrecy would vanish because in the supposed circumstances it would be precisely by the revelation of the professional secret that the common good would be protected.

Thus, for example, if the State, as the official custodian of the common good, considers the reporting of all gunshot wounds to police authorities as a necessary means for the effective control of crime, then the doctor has an obligation to report such wounds to the proper authorities.

Basic Principle III: The professional secret may, but need not be divulged when a patient, having lost his right to natural secrecy by becoming an unjust aggressor, is threatening harm to an innocent third party under the cover of professional secrecy.

Consider the following case: A patient has a highly contagious disease which also renders him sterile. He is going to marry a young lady, whom he refuses to inform of his condition. Moreover, his doctor is a second cousin of the intended bride. Hence the question: does the doctor have an obligation to reveal his patient's condition to the intended bride, who is also his own second cousin; and if he does not have an obligation to do so, is he permitted to do so?

Since the girl is being unjustly deprived of this information, and since it is only by possessing such knowledge that she can protect herself from an unjust aggression, it is evident that, in so far as the obligation of natural secrecy is concerned, any private individual who knows this fact has a fundamental obligation in charity to communicate it to her if he can do so without involving himself in serious difficulty. The aggressor, by his unjust aggression, has lost his right to his natural secret.

However, when the doctor-patient relationship introduces

the added note of professional secrecy, the answer is not so immediately evident.

Theological opinion is divided as to the right or obligation of the physician to reveal a professional secret in order to avert an unjust aggression from an innocent third party.

While it is clear that the aggressor has lost his right to his natural secret, it is not so clear that the obligation of professional secrecy has been dissolved.

It must be remembered that the obligations of professional secrecy are based not so much on the individual patient's right to secrecy as on the necessity of professional secrecy for the protection of the common good. And although it would seem that such a means to protect the innocent could not be construed as contrary to the common good, the opposite opinion is not without some solid probability.

Therefore, although a physician could reveal a professional secret in order to ward off unjust aggression from an innocent third party, we do not believe that he can be obliged to do so.

Some Particular Applications

Marriage Impediments: Canon 1027 of the Code of Canon Law opens a question in the field of professional secrecy which is somewhat analogous to the situation described above, and which is of great practical importance for the doctor.

Canon 1027: "All the faithful are bound, if they know of any impediment, to make known the same to the pastor or Ordinary of the Place before the celebration of marriage."

Although the physician will frequently be the first one to discover such an impediment to a contemplated marriage, and although he should certainly point out the impediment to the patient, it is at least probable in theory and therefore certain in practice that he is excused from the obligation of Canon 1027, in view of his professional status.[294]

Auto-aggression: A situation sometimes arises wherein a patient might be considered, as it were, an unjust aggressor against himself; and wherein the physician envisions a violation of professional secrecy in order to supply the patient's friend or relative with knowledge whereby the interested party can protect the patient against his own vices. The situation described here is not meant to include cases of mental illness which need custodial care, but rather looks to the case of one whose more or less vicious habits are a detriment to his own health.

Thus the question: Can a professional secret be revealed to some interested third party in order to protect the patient from his own vices?

Theologians differ on this question also. The concept of charity toward the patient certainly enters in here. However, unless the third party has some definite right to this knowledge, within the professional contract, we believe that the doctor is bound to maintain professional secrecy.

The reasons for maintaining professional secrecy in this case seem even stronger than those in the case of the ordinary unjust aggression mentioned previously. Here the patient is able to remedy his own situation, if he so wills. It certainly does not seem that charity demands a weakening of the bulwark of professional secrecy in order to extricate someone from a situation from which, absolutely speaking, he can extricate himself.

In this and other cases of doubtful obligation to reveal some professional knowledge, although the doctor can act on the principles of probabilism and adopt the more lenient view in favor of revelation of the secret, we believe his inclination should be in favor of maintaining professional secrecy.

Professional Secrecy and the Third Party Contract: There are certain circumstances in which, from the nature of the case, a third party enters into the professional secrecy situation, not just as an interested party, but actually as a party to the contract. Such a third party may have a right to all or only part of the matter protected by professional secrecy. These circumstances are verified in the following instances:

Infants: Parents or lawful guardians have a right to all of the professional information which the doctor has gained in treatment of children who are under the age of seven years, or who have not attained the use of reason. This would be likewise true in the case of those who are insane to such a degree that they can be said to completely lack the use of reason. All such are technically classified as "infants."

Children: Children who have attained the use of reason, but have not yet reached the age of legal adulthood, unless such children have become "emancipated" by marrying or entering the religious life, are still under parental direction and control, but not to the same extent as infants.

If such a child is sent to the physician by his parents, the physician becomes the agent of the parents in the fulfillment of their duty to protect and safeguard the child. As such an agent, the doctor must submit to the parents or guardians whatever findings result from the examination of the child. However, information which such a minor patient volunteers and which would be a natural secret should be considered to be protected by the additional right of professional secrecy.

Other Cases of Agency: Sometimes the doctor will find himself in the position of acting as medical agent for some moral person or corporation to which the patient is subject, either by his own will or in some other legitimate way.

Such would be the case when an individual agrees to have a medical examination before taking out insurance, before entering some voluntary organization such as a religious order, or before voluntary or conscripted military service.

In such circumstances the physician should keep in mind both the purpose of the physical examination and the amount of detail in his report which will be required to fulfill this purpose, and then limit his report strictly to these matters.

When the patient is seeking voluntarily to associate himself with an organization, and there are contraindicating elements in the doctor's findings, the doctor should so advise the patient, if possible. In this way an opportunity is offered to the patient simply to withdraw his application without suffering the revelation of the physician's findings.

Members of Religious Institutes: A man or woman who has entered a Religious Institute has voluntarily limited the exercise of certain human and legal rights in the interest of a greater good, and has entered into a relationship with his religious superiors which is both paternal and administrative. The former (paternal) is confined to what is called the "internal forum" and is concerned with a fatherly solicitude and care for the individual, while the latter (administrative) looks to the external government of the Institute in its corporate work. Of course, in the day to day life of the Religious Institute, these two spheres of activity often overlap and are sometimes indistinguishable.

Since, in this context, the Religious has devoted his abilities and potential to the corporate work of the Institute, and in turn the Institute supplies all of his needs (including medical care), it is understood that the Superior is party to the professional contract. He has a right to be informed of the subject's state of health and prognosis, in view of the administrative and paternal roles which the subject has freely accepted by voluntarily asking to become a member of the Institute. -

This right, however, while it extends to all ordinary health reports and therapeutic measures, is not an unlimited right. It does not extend to any invasion of privacy concerning the subject's moral conscience, his inner feelings and desires, or his hidden moral transgressions. While the subject is free to impart such information to the Superior, and is even encouraged to be thus open with him, the Superior is forbidden, by the Code of Canon Law (Canon 530) to exact such information in any way. Moreover, if the subject gives him this type of information "in the internal forum," the Superior can use it only in his paternal, and not his administrative role.

Hence the physician should remember that if a member of a Religious Institute reveals matter protected by this area of privacy, whether in interviews or in psychometric tests which he has been told to undergo, such matter may be discussed with no one other than the patient himself, without the patient's consent. And even when, with the patient's consent, the physician makes a report to the Superior in matters of such personal privacy, it would be appropriate to indicate that it is meant for the internal forum only.

In the event that administrative action by the Superior would be urgently demanded to avert an imminent and grave threat to the common good, the ordinary norms for revelation of the secret would apply. But if, by chance (e.g., in a theopental sodium interview with a priest), a physician came into possession of material protected by the seal of confession, it could not be revealed under any circumstances whatever, since nothing could be more dangerous to the common good than such a revelation.

Professional Secrets and the Civil Law: Civil law in the United States is based mainly on the English Common Law, except where changes have been introduced by particular statute.

The English Common Law did not protect the medical secret. The violation of the secret was not punished by the law itself, nor was the physician granted exemption from testifying in court.

> *English Common Law:* A medical practitioner, when called as a witness, is bound, if asked, and if the question is pressed and allowed, to disclose every communication, however private and confidential, which has been made to him while attending a patient in his professional character.[295]

Many of the individual states of the United States have changed this legal attitude toward the medical secret by statutory law. The first instance of this was the New York Statute of 1828, which is quoted here because it has been the model of subsequent statutory law in many other states:

> *New York Statute:* A person duly authorized to practice physic or surgery, or a professional or registered nurse, shall not be allowed to disclose any information which he acquired in attending a patient in a professional capacity, and which was necessary to enable him to act in that capacity; unless the patient is a child under the age of sixteen, the information so acquired indicates that the patient has been the witness or the subject of a crime, in which cases the physician or nurses may be required to testify fully in relation thereto upon any examination, trial, or other proceeding in which the commission of such crimes is subject of inquiry.[296]

The details of the statutory legislation of the several states are the subject matter of Medical Jurisprudence. The above is meant only to give some general idea of the matter of professional secrecy as it stands in the civil law.

It should be noted, however, that hospital records, in so far as they disclose what a physician has learned in attending a given case, are considered privileged communications. The privilege is considered waived when a patient sues a physician for alleged malpractice, or when the patient himself freely testifies regarding professional communications, or calls his physician as a witness.[297] Moreover, the same respect for the confidential information regarding the patient should extend to tissue reports and sections and these should not be released to another hospital or physician without the permission of the patient.[298] Although evidence obtained at autopsy is not legally privileged, since a dead body is not a patient, the moral obligation of natural secrecy will sometimes put limits to the use of information obtained at autopsy.

Professional Secrecy and Ecclesiastical Law: In connection with the moral aspects of the professional secret, it is interesting to note the extensive protection of such secrets in the ecclesiastical courts, as provided for explicitly in the Code of Canon Law:

Canon 1707: "Witnesses legitimately questioned by the judge must answer and tell the truth. Besides the priest and others who have knowledge of sacramental confessions (Cf. canon 1757, par. 3, b.) the following persons are exempted from the obligation to answer:

1. Pastors and other priests in connection with those matters which have been made known to them by reason of the sacred ministry outside of sacramental confession; civil magistrates, physicians, midwives, lawyers, notaries, and others who are also bound to official secrecy by reason of advice given in reference to affairs connected with this secret. . .

General Obligation to Inform of Negative Prognosis

In addition to the specific service of indicating the appropriate time for the administration of the sacraments for the Catholic patient, there is question of the general obligation of a physician to help the patient become aware of impending death.

This does not mean, of course, that a physician is bound personally to inform each of his critical patients that death is approaching. In many cases the patient and the patient's relatives will gradually become aware of the terminal nature of the illness, and will recognize the situation in due time.

In other cases the doctor may diagnose a fatal disease in a patient with a life expectancy of many months, and may feel that to inform this particular patient of the situation at this time would be really to the detriment of the patient. Certainly such delicate circumstances require careful timing and prudent reserve.

But a situation sometimes arises in which a doctor sees that it would be greatly to the overall spiritual and/or material advantage of his patient to give him a true picture of his prognosis, either explicitly, or at least implicitly and by suggestion.

The obligation to act at such a time can be very serious, particularly if the patient would incur serious loss, either materially or spiritually, if not informed.

Legal Aspect: The civil law tends to support this obligation. Note the following legal commentary on this type of situation:

> It is extremely unlikely that, in any ordinary circumstances, a court will find that a therapeutic privilege exists which permits a physician to withhold a specific diagnosis from a patient sick with serious or fatal illness. Unless the patient himself indicates a desire to the contrary, it appears to be clear that the confidential relationship requires that the physician make a frank and full disclosure to his adult, mentally competent patient of all the pertinent facts of the case. Any individual may soundly maintain his right to make his own decisions and that concealment of the diagnosis from his knowledge has prevented him from intelligently deciding upon a course of action.[299]

Professional Aspect: The ethical directives of the American Medical Association are explicit on this subject. In the following quotation we find the accepted professional procedure in circumstances of terminal illness:

> The physician should neither exaggerate nor minimize the gravity of the patient's condition. He should assume himself that the patient's relatives or his responsible friends have such knowledge of the patient's condition as will serve the best interests of the patient and the family.[300]

Moral Aspect: The moral obligation sometimes to assist the patient in achieving an awareness of his critical condition is stressed by the theologians and reflected in the Ethical and Religious Directives for Catholic Health Facilities as follows:

Everyone has the right and the duty to prepare for the solemn moment of death. Unless it is clear, therefore, that a dying patient is already well-prepared for death as regards both spiritual and temporal affairs, it is the physician's duty to inform him of his critical condition or to have some other responsible person impart this information. (Directive 8).

NOTES

1. Farnsworth, Dana L., writing in *To Live and To Die*, ed. by R. H. Williams, (New York, Springer-Verlag, 1973).
2. *Humanistic Perspectives in Medical Ethics*, ed. by Maurice Visscher, (Prometheus Books, 1972), p. 163.
3. Excerpts from the statement issued by the Bishops of the United States, Nov. 18, 1951. "God's Law: Measure of Man's Conduct." *The Catholic Mind*, (Feb., 1952), pp. 121ff.
4. Vatican II, *Gaudium et Spes*, par. 3.
5. Ibid.
6. Vatican I, of H. Denziger, ed. C. Banwart, ed. J. Umberg, *Enchiridion Symbolorum*, 24-25 ed., (Barcelona, 1948), no. 1839.
7. Vatican II, *Lumen Gentium*, no. 25.
8. Ibid.
9. Pius XII, Radio Message on the Education of The Christian Conscience, *Acta Apostolicae Sedis*, vol. 44, (1952), p. 275.
10. Aquinas, Thomas, *Summa Theologica*, 1a, 2ae, 91, 2.
11. Vatican II, *Gaudium et Spes*, par. 79.
12. Fuchs, Josef, *Natural Law*, (New York, Sheed and Ward, 1965), ch. 7.
13. Code of Canon Law, canon 12.
14. Aquinas, Thomas, *Summa Theologica*, 1a, 2ae, pp. 18-21.
15. Fletcher, Joseph, writing in *To Live and To Die*, ed. by Robert H. Williams, (New York, Springer-Verlag, 1973), p. 119.
16. A notable exception to the above analysis of immediate material cooperation can be had in certain cases of theft. This is because the action might be "theft" for the principal agent, while the same action might not be "theft" for the immediate material cooperator.

For example: John wishes to steal Bertha's jewelry, and because it is too heavy for him to carry alone, he forces James, at gun point, to carry the jewels away with him. In this case both men place the act together—immediate material cooperation—but while removing the jewelry is theft for John, it is not theft for James. Since, if James refused, he would lose his life, one cannot say that Bertha is "reasonably unwilling" that he should remove her property here and now.

The same reasoning would not apply in other cases because, although to remove the property of another in order to save one's life does make the act cease to be a "theft," to perform an abortion, for example, at gun point, does not make the act cease to be "abortion."

17. Public Law 93-45.

18. Pius XII, Address to the First International Congress on the Histopathology of the Nervous System. (Sept. 14, 1952).

19. DeLiguori, Alphonsus, Theologia Moralis, 1. III, no. 372.

20. DeLugo, John, De Jure et Justitia, (Lyons, 1670), disp. 10, no. 21.

21. Ballerini, Antonio—Palmieri, Dominic, Opus Theologicum Morale, (1890), vol. II, p. 614.

22. Bucceroni, Januarius, Theologia Moralis, (6th ed., 1914), vol. I, nos. 715-716.

23. Ferreres, John, Compendium Theologiae Moralis, (13th ed., 1925), vol. I, no. 349.

24. Colli-Lanzi, C., Theologia Moralis, (1928), vol. III, no. 1564.

25. Aertnys, Batavius, (ed. Damen), Theologia Moralis, 15th ed., (Brussells, 1944), vol. I, no. 566.

26. Capellmann, C., Medicina Pastoralis, 5th ed., (1901), p. 24.

27. Ibid., p. 20.

28. Konlings, A., Theologia Moralis, 5th ed., (1901), p. 24. (earliest edition at time of writing).

29. Noldin, H., Summa Theologiae Moralis, 14th ed., (1922), vol. II, no. 326.

30. Noldin, H., ed. A. Schmitt, Summa Theologiae Moralis, 27th ed., (1941), vol. II, no. 328.

31. Jone, Herbert, (translated and adapted by Adelman, German ed., (1937) and (Westminster, Md., 1953), from 13th German ed., (1949), no. 210. Hereafter, "Jone-Adelman" refers to revised edition, (Westminster, Md., 1953).

32. Lehmkuhl, Augustine, Theologia Moralis, 19th ed., (1902), vol. nos. 571-572.

33. Jone-Adelman, loc. cit.

34. Bonnar, A., The Catholic Doctor, 2nd ed., (New York, 1941), p. 96.

35. McAllister, Joseph B., Ethics, 2nd ed., (Philadelphia, 1955), p. 175.

36. DeLugo, op. cit., disp. XVI, no. 152.

37. Healy, E. F., Moral Guidance, (Chicago, 1942), p. 162.

38. Donovan, Joseph P., Homiletic and Pastoral Review, XLIX, (Aug. 1949), p. 904.

39. Kelly, Gerald, Theological Studies, XI, (June, 1950), p. 218.

40. Sullivan, Joseph V., "Catholic Teaching on the Morality of Euthanasia," Catholic University Studies in Sacred Theology, (Washington, D. C., 1949), p. 72.

41. The Jehovah's Witnesses owe their origin to Charles Taze Russell, a native of Pittsburgh, who was influenced by the second Adventists (an offshoot of the New England Mormons). The sect has opposed participation in politics, jury duty, military service, salute to the flag, vaccination and blood transfusion as being contrary to various injunctions of scripture.

42. Supreme Court of the State of New Jersey, no. a 158, September Term, 1963.

43. Roe vs. Wade; Doe vs. Bolton, (Jan. 22, 1973). Dietrick vs. Northampton, 138, Mass. 14, (1884).

44. J.A.M.A., vol. 188, no. 9, (June 1, 1964), p. 832.

45. Southworth, H., "Cardiorespiratory Resuscitation.", American Journal of Medicine, vol. 26, no. 3, (March, 1959), pp. 327-330.

46. Connery, J. R., "Current Theology.", Theological Studies, vol. 20, no. 4, (Dec., 1959), p. 607. Medical opinion indicates that cerebral anoxia of very brief duration may be sustained without damage; that up to three minutes, damage may be slight and hopefully reversible; and that after more than five minutes, under ordinary circumstances, damage is presumed to be extensive and irreversible. These periods may be lengthened under some conditions, such as intense cold or hypothermia. cf. Holser, R. M., A Manual of Cardiac Resuscitation, (Springfield, 1954).

47. Courville, C. B., Contributions to the Study of Cerebral Anoxia, (Los Angeles, 1953), p. 42.

48. Pius XII, "Address to a Symposium of the International Congress of Anesthesiology," (Nov. 24, 1957), L'Osservatore Romano, (Nov. 25-26, 1957).

49. Ibid.

50. Pius XII, Address to the First International Congress on the Histopathology of the Nervous System, (Sept. 14, 1952).

51. Pius XI, Encyclical Letter Casti Connubii, (Rome, Dec. 31, 1930).

52. Saint Thomas, Summa Theologica, IIa, IIae, Q. 65, a. 1.

53. L'Osservatore Romano, (Oct. 10, 1953).

55. Connell, Francis, American Ecclesiastical Review, CXVI, (1947), pp. 143-144.

56. Kelly, Gerald, "Medical-Moral Notes," The Linacre Quarterly, XX, no. 4, (Nov., 1953), pp. 116-117.

57. Ficarra, Bernard J., Newer Ethical Problems in Medicine and Surgery, (Westminster, Md., 1951), pp. 15-16.

58. Kelly, Gerald, Medico-Moral Problems, (St. Louis, 1957), p. 259.

59. Amelar, Richard D., "Carcinoma of the Penis due to Trauma occurring in a male patient circumcised at birth," The Journal of Urology, vol. 75, no. 4, (April, 1956), p. 728.

60. Wynder, E. L., Mantel, N., and Liklider, S. D., "Statistical Considerations on Circumcision and Cervical Cancer.", American Journal of Ob. and Gyn., vol. 79, no. 5, (May, 1960), pp. 1026-1030.

61. Opinions and Reports of the Judicial Council, Chicago, The American Medical Association, (1965), sec. 1, no. 8.

62. Bulletin of the American College of Surgeons, vol. 39, no. 2, (March-April, 1954), p. 72.

63. Ibid.

64. *Bull. Amer. Coll. Surg.*, vol. 39, no. 4, (July-Aug., 1954), p. 152.
65. Hawley, Paul R., "Redefining the Indefinable," *Bull. Amer. Coll. Surg.*, vol. 40, no. 5, (Sept.-Oct., 1955), p. 302.
66. *Opinions and Reports of the Judicial Council*, ibid.
67. Connell, Francis J., "Delegated Surgical Procedures," *Amer. Eccles. Rev.*, vol. CXXXV, no. 3, (Sept., 1956), pp. 197-198.
68. Lynch, John J., "The Resident Surgeon and the Private Patient," *The Linacre Quarterly*, vol. 23, no. 4, (Nov., 1956), pp. 117-122.
69. This analysis of the prefrontal area is drawn mainly from: Porteus, S. D. and Dpner, R., "Mental Changes after Bilateral Prefrontal Lobotomy," *Genetic Psychology* Monographs, (1944), XXIX, pp. 1-144; and from: W. Freeman, and Watts, J., *Psychosurgery* (Baltimore, 1942).
70. Sweet, W. H., "Treatment of Medically Intractable Mental Disease by Limited Frontal Leucotomy—Justifiable?", *New England Journal of Medicine*, vol. 289, (1973), pp. 1117-1124.
71. *Hastings Center Report*, Special Supplement, (May, 1973).
72. Pius XII, "Pathologists," (as above).
73. *Medical World News*, (April 9, 1965), pp. 43-45.
74. American Medical Association, "Supplementary Report of the Judicial Committee, House of Delegates, (Dec., 1946)," *J.A.M.A.*, CXXXII, 17, (Dec. 28, 1946), p. 1090.
75. Ibid.
76. Pius XII, "Allocution to the Participants of the Eighth Congress of the World Medical Association," (Sept. 30, 1954). *The Pope Speaks*, I, 4, (1954), pp. 347-359.
77. This conference (May 27-29, 1959) was sponsored by the National Society for Medical Research and the University of Chicago. Proceedings of the conference have been published by the National Society for Medical Research, (Chicago, 1959).
78. Kevorkian, J., "Capital Punishment or Capital Gain?", *Journal of Criminal Law, Criminology and Police Science, vol.* 50, (1959), pp. 50-57. See also, by the same author: *Medical Research and the Death Penalty: A Dialogue*, (New York, Vantage Press, 1960).
79. St. Thomas, *Summa Contra Gentiles*, 1, III, C. CXII.
80. Pius XII, "Address to a Group of Eye Specialists and Delegates of The Italian Association of Donors of the Cornea," (May 14, 1956). *The Pope Speaks* (Autumn, 1956), pp. 198-206. Hereafter referred to as "Pius XII, to Eye Specialists."
81. Reemtsma, K., et al., "Reversal of Early Graft Rejection After Renal Heterotransplantation in Man.", *J.A.M.A.*, vol. 187, no. 10, (March 7, 1964), pp. 691-696.
82. Pius XII, to Eye Specialists.
83. Pius XII, to Italian Assoc. of Blood Donors, (March 8, 1959), *The Pope Speaks*, vol. 5, no. 3, (Summer 1959), p. 334.

84. Connery, John R., "Notes on Moral Theology," *Theological Studies,* vol. 17, no. 4, (Dec. 1956), pp. 559-561.

85. Kelly, Gerald, "Pope Pius XII and the Principle of Totality," *Theol. Stud.,* vol. 16, no. 3, (Sept., 1955), pp. 373-396.

86. Copeland, Murray M., *et. al., The Bulletin—Georgetown University Medical Center,* VII, 3, (Jan., 1954), p. 80.

87. Miller, H. K., "Cancer of the Breast During Pregnancy Lactation." *Amer. Journ. of Ob. and Gyn.,* vol. 83, no. 5, (March 1, 1962), pp. 539ff.

88. Brooks, M. B.; Lytton, B. and Weiss, S., "Vasectomy in the Control of Epididymitis after Prostatectomy Following Urethral Catheter Drainage." *Journal of Urology,* 105, (May, 1971), p. 694.

89. Te Linde, Richard W., *Operative Gynecology,* 2nd ed., (Philadelphia, 1953), pp. 539ff.

90. Movak, Emil, and Novak, Edmund, *Textbook of Gynecology,* 5th ed., (Baltimore: Williams and Wilkins, 1956), p. 397.

91. Welch, John S., "The Surgical Treatment of Uterine Myomas in the Young Women." *The Surgical Clinics of North America,* (Aug., 1957), pp. 1101-1106.

92. *J.A.M.A.,* vol. 164, no. 3, (May 18, 1957), p. 355.

93. Lordaro, H. H., "Extensive Myomectomy." *Amer. Jour. of Ob. and Gyn.,* vol. 79, no. 1, (Jan. 1960), pp. 43-51.

94. Feroze, R. M., "Endometriosis," *Postgraduate Medical Journal,* vol. 32, (Nov., 1956), pp. 532-536.

95. Beecham, Clayton T., "Surgical Treatment of Endometriosis," *J.A.M.A.,* vol. 139, no. 15, (April 9, 1949), pp. 971-976.

96. Gray, L. A., "The Conservative Operation for Endometriosis: A report of its use in 200 Cases.", *Journ. of the Kentucky Medical Association,* vol. 58, (Dec. 1958), pp. 1219-1225.

97. Kistner, Tobert W., "The Use of Newer Progestins in the Treatment of Endometriosis," *Amer. Journ. of Ob. and Gyn.,* vol. 75, no. 2, (Feb., 1958), pp. 264-377.

98. Lebherz, T. B., and Fobes, C. D., "Management of Endometriosis with Nor-progesterone.", *Amer. Jour. of Ob. and Gyn.,* vol. 81, no. 1, (Jan., 1961), pp. 102-108.

99. Wharton, L. R., "Indications for Hysterectomy in Benign Conditions Near Menopause," *Southern Medical Journal,* no. 40, (Dec., 1957), p. 1914.

100. Conger, G. T., and Keettel, W. C., "The Manchester-Fothergill Operation, Its Place in Gynecology," *Amer. Journ. of Ob. and Gyn.,* vol. 76, no. 3, (Sept., 1958), p. 635.

101. Te Linde, R. W., *Operative Gynecology,* (Philadelphia, 1956), p. 457.

102. Te Linde, R. W., and Wharton, L. R., Jr., "Ovarian Function Following Pelvic Operation." *Amer. Journ. of Ob. and Gyn.,* vol. 80, no. 6, (Dec., 1960), pp. 1085-1088.

103. Novak, E. R., and Williams, T. J., "Autopsy Comparison of Cardiovascular Changes in Castrated and Normal Women.", *Amer. Journ. of Ob. and Gyn.*, vol. 80, no. 5, (Nov., 1960), pp. 863-869.

104. Narvekar, M. R., "Labor Following Previous Caesarean Sections," *Journ. Obst. and Gynaec.*, India, 7, pp. 115-133 (Dec., 1956).

105. Reported in *Amer. Journ. of Ob. and Gyn.*, vol. 70, no. 1, (July, 1955), p. 91.

106. A published opinion of E. Tesson likewise supports this view of *Cahier Laennec*, vol. 24, no. 6, (June, 1964), pp. 64-73.

107. Pius XII, address to The National Congress of the Family Front, (Nov., 1951).

108. Aten, P., "Legal Abortion in Sweden," *Acta Ob. et Gyn. Scandinavica*, 37, suppl. 1, (1958).

109. Tietze, C., and Lehfeld, H., "Legal Abortion in Eastern Europe." *J.A.M.A.*, vol. 175, no. 13, (April 1, 1961), pp. 1149-1153.

110. Code of Canon Law, canon 19,

111. Huser, Roger J., *The Crime of Abortion in Canon Law*, (Washington, 1942).

112. Merkelbach, Benedict, *Quaestiones de Embryologia et Sterilizatione*, (Liege, 1937), pp. 24-29.

113. Towers, Bernard, "Man in Modern Science," *The Month*, 31, 1, (Jan., 1964), pp. 25-36.

114. Migne, J.-P., *Pat. Graec.* XXXII.

115. Pius XI, *Casti Connubii*, (as above).

116. Pius XII, Allocution to Large Families, (Nov. 27, 1951).

117. John XXIII, Encyclical Letter *Mater et Magistra*, (May 15, 1961).

118. Paul VI, address to Members of the New England Obstetrical and Gynecological Society, (Oct. 3, 1964).

119. Cunningham, T. P., "The Contumacy Required to Incur Censures," *Irish Theological Quarterly*, 4, (1954), pp. 332-356.

120. This symposium was reported in the *San Francisco News* and the *Call Bulletin*, (Nov. 9, 1951).

121. Good, F. L., and Kelly, D., *Marriage, Morals and Medical Ethics*, (New York, 1951), pp. 148-149.

122. Heffernan, R. J., and Lynch, W. A., *Amer. Journ. of Ob. and Gyn.*, vol. 66, no. 2, (Aug., 1953), pp. 335-345.

123. Titus, op. cit., p. 780.

124. Eastman, N. J., ed. Williams, *Obstetrics*, 11th ed., (New York, 1956), pp. 1155-1156.

125. Cunningham, op. cit., p. 442.

126. Davis, C. H., and Carter, B., *Gynecology and Obstetrics*, (Hagerstown, 1953), vol. II, p. 65.

127. Titus, op. cit., pp. 785-786.

128. Shider, H. M., "Pregnancy Complicated by Addison's Disease.", "*Amer. Journ. of Ob. and Gyn.*", vol. 78, no. 4, (Oct. 1959), pp. 808-811;

and also Schartum, S., *Tidsskr. Norske Laegefor.*, vol. 79 (March 15, 1959), pp. 355-337.
129. Pius XI, *Casti Connubii*, (as above).
130. Montgomery, T. L., "Detection and Disposal of Breast Cancer in Pregnancy.", *Amer. Journ. of Ob. and Gyn.*, vol. 81, no. 5, (May, 1961), pp. 926-933.
131. Cheek, J. A., "Survey of Current Opinion Concerning Carcinoma of the Breast During Pregnancy.", *A.M.A. Archives of Surgery*, vol. 66, no. 5, (May, 1953), pp. 664-672.
132. Brown, R. N., "Carcinoma of the Breast Followed by Pregnancy.", *Surgery*, vol. 48, no. 5, (Nov., 1960), pp. 862-868.
133. Holleb, A. I., and Farrow, J. H., "Relation of Carcinoma of Breast and Pregnancy in 283 Cases.", *Surg., Gynec. Obstet.*, vol. 115, no. 5, (July, 1962).
134. Byrd, B. F. Jr., Bayer, D. S., Robertson, J. C., and Stephenson, S. E. Jr., "Treatment of Breast Tumors Associated with Pregnancy and Lactation.", *Annals of Surgery*, vol. 155, no. 6, (June, 1962), pp. 940-947.
135. Bunker, M. L., and Peters, M. V., "Breast Cancer Associated with Pregnancy and Lactation.", *Amer. Journ. of Ob. and Gyn.*, vol. 85, no. 3, (Feb. 1, 1963), pp. 312-321.
136. Ayre, J. E., and Scott, J. W., "Carcinoma in situ and Pregnancy.", *J.A.M.A.*, vol. 167, no. 2, (April 15, 1961), pp. 102-105.
137. Stone, M. L., Weingold, A. B., and Small, S., "Cervical Carcinoma in Pregnancy.", *Amer. Journ. of Ob. and Gyn.*, vol. 93, no. 4, (Oct. 15, 1965), pp. 479-485.
138. Kinch, R., "Factors Affecting the Prognosis of Cancer of the Cervix in Pregnancy.", *Amer. Journ. of Ob. and Gyn.*, vol. 82, no. 1, (July, 1961), pp. 45-51.
139. O'Leary, J. A., and Bepko, F. J., "Rectal Carcinoma and Pregnancy.", *Amer. Journ. of Ob. and Gyn.*, vol. 84, no. 4, (Aug. 15, 1962), pp. 459-461.
140. Warren, R., "Carcinoma of the Rectum and Pregnancy.", *British Journal of Surgery*, vol. 45, no. 189, (July, 1958), pp. 61-67.
141. Hindlemann, L., and Mestel, A. L., "Multiple Carcinomatosis of the Colon Complicating Pregnancy.", *Obstetrics and Gynecology*, vol. II, no. 2, (Jan., 1958), pp. 119-122.
142. Gorenberg, H., "Rheumatic Heart Disease, A Controllable Complication of Pregnancy.", *Amer. Journ. of Ob. and Gyn.*, vol. XLV, no. 5, (May, 1943), p. 835.
143. O'Driscoll, M. K., Coyle, F., and Drury, M., "Rheumatic Heart Disease Complicating Pregnancy.", *British Medical Journal*, vol. 2, no. 5307, (Sept. 1962), pp. 767-768.
144. Burwell, C. Sidney, "The Special Problem of Rheumatic Heart Disease in Pregnant Women," *J.A.M.A.*, vol. 166, no. 2, (Jan. 11, 1958), pp. 153-158.

145. Winter, William R., et al., "Cardiac Surgery Associated With Pregnancy," *Amer. Journ. of Ob. and Gyn.*, vol. 90, no. 1, (Sept. 1, 1964), pp. 73-77.

146. Burt, R. L., and Bowden, R. H., Jr., "Pregnancy Following Cardiac Surgery.", *Amer. Journ. of Ob. and Gyn*, vol. 90, no. 1, (Sept. 1, 1964), pp. 73-77.

147. Adams, J. Q., and Cameron, W. B., "The Management of Eclampsia.", *Amer. Journ of Ob. and Gyn.*, vol. 80, no. 2, (Aug., 1960), pp. 253-257.

148. Page, Ernest W., "Functions of the Human Placenta.", *Modern Medicine*, vol. 28, no. 3, (Feb. 1, 1960), pp. 26-32.

149. McReavy, L. L., "Eclampsia and Abortion," *The Clergy Review*, vol. XLIV, no. 3, (March, 1959), pp. 180-183. Connery, John R., "Current Theology," *Theological Studies*, vol. 20, no. 4, (Dec., 1959), pp. 603-604.

150. Berger, Max, and Cavanagh, Denis, "Toxemia of Pregnancy," *Amer. Journ. of Ob. and Gyn.*, vol. 87, no. 3, (Oct., 1961), pp. 293-305.

151. Bartholomew, R. A., et al., "Facts Pertinent to the Etiology of Eclamptogenic Toxemia.", *Amer. Journ. of Ob. and Gyn.*, vol. 74, no. 1, (July, 1957), pp. 64-84.

152. Cunningham, J. F., *Textbook of Obstetrics*, (London, 1951), p. 140.

153. *J.A.M.A.*, "References and Reviews.", vol. 172, no. 11, (March 12, 1960), p. 1206.

154. McClure, J. H., "Idiopathy Epilepsy in Pregnancy.", *Amer. Journ. of Ob. and Gyn.*, vol. 7, no. 2, (Aug., 1955), pp. 296-301.

155. Janz and Fuchs, "Are Anti-Epileptic Drugs Harmful During Pregnancy?", *La Clinica Ginecologica*, vol. 4, no. 6, (1962), p. 24.

156. Bevis, D. C. A., "Antenatal Prediction of Hemolytic Disease of the Newborn,", *Lancet*, vol. 1, no. 6704, (Feb. 23, 1952), pp. 395-398.

157. Liley, A. W., "Intrauterine Transfusion of Fetus in Hemolytic Disease.", *British Medical Journal*, vol. 2, no. 5365, (Nov. 2, 1963), pp. 1107-1109.

158. Freda, V. J., and Adamsons, K. Jr., "Exchange Transfusion in Utero.", *Amer. Journ. of Ob. and Gyn.*, vol. 89, no. 6, (July 15, 1964), pp. 817-821.

159. Bowes, W. A. Jr., Drose, V. E., and Bruns, P. D., "Amniocentesis and Intrauterine Fetal Transfusion in Erythroblastosis.", *Amer. Journ. of Ob. and Gyn.*, vol. 93, no. 6, (Nov. 15, 1965), pp. 822-837.

160. Heffernan and Lynch, *The Linacre Quarterly*, loc. cit.

161. Hoja, W. J., "Gaucher's Disease in Pregnancy.", *Amer. Journ. of Ob. and Gyn.*, vol. 79, no. 2, (Feb., 1960), pp. 286-293.

162. Ryrie, G. A., "Pregnancy and Leprosy.", *British Medical Journal*, vol. 2, no. 4043, (July 2, 1938), p. 39.

163. King, J. A., and Marks, R. A., "Pregnancy and Leprosy.", *Amer. Journ. of Ob. and Gyn.*, vol. 76, no. 2, (Aug., 1958), pp. 438-441.

164. Long, J. S., Boyson, H., and Priest, F. O., "Infectious Hepatitis and Pregnancy.", *Amer. Journ. of Ob. and Gyn.*, vol. 70, no. 2, (Aug., 1955), pp. 282-288.

165. Adams, R. H., and Combes, B., "Viral Hepatitis During Pregnancy," *J.A.M.A.*, vol. 192, no. 3, (April 19, 1965), pp. 195-198.

166. Barry, R. M., and Craver, L. F., "Influence of Pregnancy on the Course of Hodgkin's Disease.", *Amer. Journ of Ob. and Gyn.*, vol. 84, no. 4, (Aug. 15, 1962), pp. 445-454.

167. Hennessy, J. P., and Rottino, A., "Hodgkin's Disease in Pregnancy.", *Amer. Journ. of Ob. and Gyn.*, vol. 87, no. 7, (Dec. 1, 1963), pp. 851-853.

168. Titus, *op. cit.*, p. 276.

169. Rubin, I. C., and Novak, Josef, *Integrated Gynecology*, (New York, 1956), vol. II, p. 196.

170. *Amer. Journ of Ob. and Gyn.*, vol. 79, no. 5, (May, 1960), vol. 79, no. 6, (June, 1960), vol. 88, no. 6, (Nov. 15, 1964).

171. Tancer, M. L., "Idiopathic Thrombocytopenic Purpura and Pregnancy.", *Amer. Journ. of Ob. and Gyn.*, vol. 79, no. 1, (Jan., 1960), pp. 148-153.

172. Dugan, P. J., and Black, M. E., "Kyphoscoliosis and Pregnancy.", *Amer. Journ. of Ob. and Gyn.*, vol. 73, no. 1, (Jan., 1957), pp. 89-93.

173. Lee, R. A., Johnson, C. E., and Hanlon, D. G., "Leukemia During Pregnancy.", *Amer. Journ. of Ob. and Gyn.*, vol. 84, no. 4, (Aug. 15, 1962), pp. 455-458.

174. Mulla, N., "Acute Leukemia and Pregnancy.", *Amer. Journ. of Ob. and Gyn.*, vol. 75, no. 6, (June, 1958), pp. 1283-1285.

175. Donaldson, L. B., and deAlverez, R. L., "Further Observations on Lupus Erythematosus Associated with Pregnancy,", *Amer. Journ. of Ob. and Gyn.*, vol. 83, no. 11, (June 1, 1962), pp. 1461-1471.

176. Dziubinski, E. H., Winkelmann, R. K., and Wilson, R. B., "Systemic Lupus Erythematosus and Pregnancy.", *Amer. Journ. of Ob. and Gyn.*, vol. 84, no. 12, (Dec. 15, 1962), pp. 1873-1877.

177. Friedman, E. A., and Rutherford, J. W., "Pregnancy and Lupus Erythematosus.", *Obstetrics and Gynecology*, vol. 8, no. 5, (Nov., 1956), pp. 601-610.

178. Sweeney, W. J., "Pregnancy and Multiple Sclerosis.", *Clinical Obstetrics and Gynecology*, vol. 1, no. 1, (March, 1958), pp. 137-145.

179. Garvin, J. S., "Multiple Sclerosis and Pregnancy.", *Amer. Journ. of Ob. and Gyn.*, vol. 83, no. 5, (March 1, 1962), pp. 689-699.

180. Plauche, W. C., "Myasthenia Gravis in Pregnancy.", *Amer. Journ. of Ob. and Gyn.*, vol. 88, no. 3, (Feb. 1, 1964), pp. 404-409.

181. *J.A.M.A.*, "Foreign Letters," vol. 174, no. 7, (Oct. 15, 1960), p. 909.

182. Overstreet, E. W., and Trout, H. F., "Indications for Therapeutic Abortion," *Post-Graduate Medicine*, vol. 9, no. 10, (Oct. 1951), pp. 16-25.

183. Fulty, G. S. Jr., "Therapeutic Abortion.", *Southern Medical Journal,* vol. 47, no. 1, (Jan., 1954), pp. 55-58.

184. Hardin Brauch, C. H., and Reiser, D. E., "Personality Reactions to Uterine Functions.", *GP,* vol. X, no. 3, (Sept., 1954), pp. 39-46.

185. Arbuse, D. I., and Schedtman, J., "Neuropsychiatric Indications for Therapeutic Abortion.", *American Practitioner,* vol. I, no. 10, (Oct., 1950), pp. 1069-1075.

186. Rosenberg, A. J., and Silver, E., "Suicide, Psychiatrists and Therapeutic Abortion.", *California Medicine,* vol. 102, no. 6, (June, 1965), pp. 704-711.

187. Haskins, A. L., "Questions and Answers.", *J.A.M.A.,* vol. 180, no. 13, (June 30, 1962), p. 1152.

188. *J.A.M.A.,* "Foreign Letters," vol. 174, no. 7, (Oct. 15, 1960), p. 909.

189. Rosenbach, L. M., and Gangemi, C. R., "Tuberculosis and Pregnancy.", *J.A.M.A.,* vol. 161, no. 11, (July 14, 1956), pp. 1035-1038.

190. Jacobs, Sidney, "Tuberculosis and Pregnancy.", *Diseases of the Chest,* vol. XXX, no. 1, (July, 1956), pp. 43-49.

191. Myers, J. A., "Questions and Answers.", *J.A.M.A.,* vol. 184, no. 6, (May 11, 1963), p. 523.

192. Brugsch, H. G., and Brodie, S., "Polycystic Kidney Disease Complicated by Pregnancy.", *Bulletin of the New England Medical Center,* vol. X, no. 5, (Oct., 1948), pp. 202-212.

193. Cunningham, op. cit., p. 159.

194. Heffernan, R. J., and Lynch, W. A., "Is Therapeutic Abortion Scientifically Justified?", *The Linacre Quarterly,* vol. XIIX, no. 1, (Feb., 1952), pp. 11-27.

195. Tenney, B., and Dandrow, R. V., "Clinical Study of Hypertensive Disease in Pregnancy.", *Amer. Journ. of Ob. and Gyn.,* vol. 81, no. 1, (Jan., 1961), pp. 8-15.

196. Herwig, K. R., Merrill, J. P., Jackson, R. L., and Oken, D. E., "Chronic Renal Disease and Pregnancy.", *Amer. Journ. of Ob. and Gyn.,* vol. 92, no. 8, (Aug. 15, 1965), pp. 1117-1121.

197. Eastman, op. cit., p. 756.

198. Editorial: "The Risks of Rubella," *GP,* X, 3, (Sept., 1954), p. 30.

199. Editorial: "Rubella and Pregnancy," *J.A.M.A.,* vol. 165, no. 6, (Oct. 12, 1957), p. 688.

200. Greenberg, Morris, Pellitteri, Ottavio, and Barton, Jerome, "Frequency of Defects in Infants Whose Mothers Had Rubella During Pregnancy." *J.A.M.A.,* vol. 165, no. 6, (Oct. 12, 1957), pp. 675-678.

201. Kantor, H. I., and Strother, W. K., "German Measles in Pregnancy.", *Amer. Journ. of Ob. and Gyn.,* vol. 81, no. 5, (May, 1961), pp. 902-905.

202. Kelly, Gerald, *Medico-Moral Problems V,* (St. Louis, 1954), p. 16.

203. McPheeters, H. O., "Value of Estrogen Therapy in Treatment of

Varicose Veins Complicating Pregnancy.", *Journal-Lancet,* vol. 69, no. 1, (Jan., 1949), pp. 2-4.

204. Nabatoff, R. A., "Varicose Veins of Pregnancy.", *J.A.M.A.,* vol. 174, no. 13, (Nov. 26, 1960), pp. 1712-1716.

205. Litzenberg, op. cit., p. 330.

206. DeLee-Grennhill, op. cit., p. 407.

207. Titus, op. cit., p. 369.

208. Marchetti, Andrew, *A Consideration of Obstetric Hemorrhage* (manuscript copy).

209. Op. cit., p. 271.

210. Eastman, op. cit., p. 489.

211. DeLee-Greenhill, op. cit., p. 337.

212. Cf. Vaish, R., "Term Tubal Pregnancy with Survival of Mother and Infant," *American Journal of Obstetrics and Gynecology,* vol. 77, no. 6, (June, 1959), p. 1309.

213. Studdiford, W. E., *Amer. Journ. of Ob. and Gyn.,* vol. 49, no. 169, (1945).

214. DeLee-Greenhill, op. cit., p. 359.

215. Good and Kelly, op. cit., p. 97.

216. Bouscaren, T. Lincoln, *Ethics of Ectopic Operations,* 2nd ed., (Milwaukee, 1944), p. 102.

217. Wallace, C. J., "Transplantations of Ectopic Pregnancy from Fallopian Tube to Cavity of Uterus," *Surgery, Gynecology, and Obstetrics,* XXIV, 5, (May, 1917), pp. 578-579.

218. Eastman, op. cit., p. 1035.

219. DeLee-Greenhill, op. cit., p. 962.

220. *J.A.M.A.,* CXLVII, 17, (Dec. 22, 1951), pp. 1719-1720.

221. Bishop, E. H., "Dangers attending elective induction of labor," *J.A.M.A.,* vol. 166, no. 16, (April 19, 1958), pp. 1953-1956.

222. Eastman, op. cit., p. 425.

223. Pius XII, Address to a Group of Catholic Obstetricians and Gynecologists, (Jan. 8, 1956), *The Pope Speaks,* vol. 3, no. 1, (Spring-Summer, 1956).

224. Gn 3:16.

225. Eastman, op. cit., p. 459.

226. Titus, op. cit., p. 992.

227. Litzenberg, op. cit., p. 132.

228. For a canonical analysis of this question cf. Cappello, F. M., *De Sacramentis,* 6th ed., (Rome, 1950), vol. V, nos. 342-349, 382.

229. Rubin and Novak, op. cit., vol. III, p. 82.

230. Ombredanne, Professor, "The Marriage of Hermaphrodites," with a Theological Note by Tesson, P., *New Problems in Medical Ethics,* ed. Dom Peter Flood, (Westminster, 1952), vol. 1, pp. 50-60.

231. Ford, John C., "Notes on Moral Theology, Marriage," *Theol. Stud.,* 5, (Dec., 1944), pp. 533-534.

232. Healy, Edwin F., op. cit., p. 137.

233. Cone, F., "A Survey of the Present Status and Problems of Sterility," *Texas State Journal of Medicine*, XXXVII, 1, (May, 1941), pp. 20-25.

234. Cliffoid, "Sterility Tests and their Morality," *Amer. Eccles. Rev.*, CIX, 5, (Nov., 1952), p. 365.

235. Charny, C. W., "Questions and Answers," *J.A.M.A.*, vol. 176, no. 7, (May 20, 1961), p. 641.

236. van Andel, J. G., "Radiological Treatment of Plastic Induration of the Penis." *Nederlands Tijdschr Geneeskunde*, vol. 108, (Dec. 5, 1964), pp. 2350-2353.

237. Gaspari, P., *Tractatus Canonicus de Matrimonio* (Rome, 1932), I, append. de vasect.

De Smet, A., *De Sponsalibus et Matrimonio*, (Bruges, 1927), no. 440.

Marc-Gesterman, op. cit., vol. II, no. 2009.

Wouters, B., *Theologia Moralis*, (Rome, 1932), vol. II, no. 774.

Tanquerey, A., *Synopsis Theologia Moralis et Pastoralis*, (Rome, 1920), vol. 1, supp. 5.

Wernz, F. X. (Vidal), *Jus Canonicum*, (Rome, 1925), vol. V, no. 233.

Cappello, F., *De Sacramentis*, (Rome, 1933), vol. III, Merkelbach, B., *Questiones de Embryologia et Sterilizatione*, (Liege, 1937), p. 93.

Bucceroni, op. cit., vol. IV, no. 63.

Ubach, J., *Compendium Theologiae Moralis*, (Freiburg, 1929), vol. II, no. 798.

238. In several cases a Roman Pontiff has granted a dissolution of the bond in a supposedly sacramental marriage when the only defect was a lack of testicular semen in the male ejaculate, in one case due to bilateral occlusion of the vasa deferentia by nodular formations. In the canonical context of such a dissolution of the bond the evident implication is that, although the defect was not certainly permanent and hence the marriage was presumed valid, carnal copula totally devoid of testicular products was not considered as a true marital act, and hence these marriages were not considered to have been consummated. (see: *Periodica*, XXXIII 216, 1944). While this type of jurisdictional act, on the part of a Pope, provides a strong argument for this view, it does not constitute a definitive papal teaching.

239. Ford, John C., "Double Vasectomy and the Impediment of Impotence.", *Theol. Stud.* XVI, 4, (1955), pp. 533-557.

240. Vermeersch, A., *Theologisch-praktische Auartalschrift*, LXXXIX (1936), 59. Jorio, T., *Theologia Moralis* (Naples, 1940), vol. III, part II, no. 1178. Noldin-Schmitt, op. cit., vol. III, no. 567. Bouscaren, T. L., and Ellis, A. C., *Canon Law, Code and Commentary*, (Milwaukee, 1945), p. 526.

241. Barr, M. L., "Cytological Tests of Sex," *Lancet*, 1, 47 (Jan. 7, 1956), p. 47.

242. Hampson, J. G., Money, J., Hampson, J. L., "Hermaphrodism. Recommendations Concerning Case Management." *Journal of Clinical Endoctrinology and Metabolism,* 16, pp. 547-556, (April, 1956).

243. Tesson, P., op. cit., p. 58.

244. Cf. a private reply of the Sacred Congregation of the Propagation of the Faith as quoted in: Bouscaren, T. L., *The Canon Law Digest,* (Milwaukee, 1934), vol. I, p. 511.

245. Pius XI, *Casti Connubii,* (as above).

246. Pius XII, Address to the Italian Catholic Union of Midwives, (Oct. 29, 1951), *Acta Apostolicae,* XLIII, pp. 835-854. Hereafter referred to simply as "Midwives."

247. Second Vatican Council, The Constitution on the Church in the Modern World, Part II, ch. I, no. 51.

248. Paul VI, Encyclical Letter "Humanae Vitae," (July 25, 1968).

249. Sieve, B. J., "A New Antifertility Factor (A Preliminary Report)," *Science, vol.* 116, no. 3015, (Oct. 10, 1952), pp. 373-385.

250. Williams, W. W., "Questions and Answers," *J.A.M.A.,* 174, 7, (Oct. 15, 1960), p. 923.

251. Salmon, M. L., Winkelman, J. Z., and Gay, A. J., "Neuro-opthalmic Sequelae in Users of Oral Contraceptives.", *J.A.M.A.,* 206, 1, (Sept. 30, 1968), pp. 85-91.

252. Wilkins, Lawson, "Masculinization of female fetus due to use of orally given progestins.", *J.A.M.A.,* 172, 10, March 5, 1960, pp. 1028-1032.

253. Wilson, J. R., et al., "The Margulies Intrauterine Contraceptive Device.", *Amer. Journ. of Ob. and Gyn.,* 29, 1, (Oct. 1, 1965), pp. 62-70; Burnhill, M. S., and Birnberg, C. H., "Uterine Perforation with Intrauterine Contraceptive Devices." *idem,* 98, 1, (May 1, 1967), pp. 135-140.

254. Wilson, J. R., Ledger, W. J., and Andros, G. J., "The Effect of an Intrauterine Contraceptive Device on the Histologic Pattern of the Endometrium.", *Amer. Journ. of Ob. and Gyn.,* 93, 6, (Nov. 15, 1965), pp. 802-811.

255. Pius XII, Address to the Italian Catholic Union of Midwives, Oct. 29, 1951, *Acta Apostolicae Sedis,* XLIII, pp. 834, 854. Also Paul VI, *Humanae Vitae,* no. 16.

256. O'Connor, V. J., "Anastomosos of Vas Deferens after Purposeful Division for Sterility," *J.A.M.A.,* CXXXVI, 3, (Jan. 17, 1948), p. 162.

257. Dorsey, J. W., "Anastomosis of the Vas Deferens to Correct Post-Vasectomy Sterility," *Journal of Urology,* 70, 3, (Sept., 1953), p. 515.

258. Schmidt, S. S., "Anastomosis of the Vas Deferens: An Experimental Study, I," *Journal of Urology,* 75, 2, (Feb., 1956), pp. 300-303.

259. Cappello, F., *De Sacramentis,* 5th ed., (Turin, 1947). V. no. 814.

260. Ibid., no. 370 d.

261. Vermeersch, op. cit., vol. IV, no. 76.

262. McFadden, op. cit., p. 97.

263. McCarthy, J., "Notes and Queries," *The Irish Ecclesiastical Rec-*

ord, fifth series, LXX, 966, (June, 1948), p. 534.

264. Tyler, E., "Semen Studies and Fertility," *J.A.M.A.,* CXLVI, 4, (May 26, 1951), pp. 307-314.

265. Viergiver, E., and Pommerenke, W., "Cyclic Variations in the Viscosity of Cervical Mucus and its Correlation with Amounts of Secretion and Basal Temperature," *Amer. Journ. of Ob. and Gyn.,* LI, 2, (Feb., 1946), pp. 192-200.

266. Doyle, J., "The Cervical Spoon . . . an Aid to Spermigration and Semen Sampling," *Bulletin of the New England Medical Center,* X, 5, (Oct., 1948), pp. 225-231.

267. Schellen, A. M. C. M., *Artificial Insemination in the Human* (Amsterdam, 1957), pp. 7-10.

268. Pius XII, Address to the Fourth International Congress of Catholic Doctors, (Sept. 29, 1949), *Discorsi e Radiomessagi,* XI (Vatican Press), pp. 221-225. Hereafter referred to simply as "Catholic Doctors."

269. Ford, John C., "Current Theology," *Theol. Stud.,* vol. 5, no. 4, (Dec., 1944), p. 513.

270. Pius XII, "Address to the Second World Congress on Fertility and Sterility," *The Pope Speaks,* (Autumn, 1956), pp. 191-197.

271. Donovan, Joseph P., "Answer to Questions," *Homiletic and Pastoral Review,* XLV, (Oct., 1944), pp. 9-60.

272. Schellen, A. M. C. M., op. cit., passim.

273. Kelly, S. J., Gerald, *Medico-Moral Problems* (St. Louis, 1957), p. 238.

274. Charny, C. W., "Treatment of Male Infertility with Large Doses of Testosterone," *J.A.M.A.,* vol. 160, no. 2, (Jan. 14, 1956), pp. 98-106.

275. Eastman, op. cit., p. 494.

276. Cunningham, op. cit., p. 449.

277. e.g., I Cor 6.

278. Levine, Milton, and Bell, Anita, I. "The Psychologic Aspects of Pediatric Practice," II. "Masturbation," *Pediatrics* 18, 5, (Nov., 1956), pp. 803-808.

279. Davis, Henry, op. cit., vol. II, p. 254; also McCarthy, John, *Irish Ecclesiastical Record,* (June, 1949), p. 548.

280. Novak, Emil, *The Woman Asks the Doctor,* 2nd ed., (Baltimore, 1944), pp. 79-80.

281. Thornton, Madeline J., "The Use of Vaginal Tampons for the Absorption of Menstrual Discharge." *Amer. Journ. of Ob. and Gyn.,* vol. 46, (Aug., 1943), pp. 259-265.

282. Kelly, Gerald, "Medical-Moral Notes," *The Linacre Quarterly,* vol. 17, no. 4, (Nov., 1950), p. 16.

283. Dickinson, R. L., "Tampons as Menstrual Guards," *J.A.M.A.,* vol. 128, no. 7, (June 16, 1945), pp. 490-494.

284. McFadden, op. cit., p. 100.

285. Vermeersch, op. cit., vol. IV., no. 79.

286. *Percival's Medical Ethics*, ed. by Chauncey Leake, (Baltimore, 1927), ch. II, no. 1.

287. *Code of Ethics of the American Medical Association*, (Philadelphia, 1848).

288. *J.A.M.A.* (Special Edition), June 7, 1958.

289. DeLugo, op. cit., disp. 14, sect. 9, no. 143.

290. Saint Thomas, *Summa Theologica*, IIa, IIae, q. 109.

291. Vermeersch, op. cit., vol. II, no. 691, 2.

292. DeLugo, loc. cit., no. 61.

293. Regan, R., *Professional Secrecy*, (Washington, 1943), p. 18.

294. Noldin-Schmitt, op. cit., vol. III, no. 550, also Bouscaren-Ellis, op. cit., p. 415.

295. Halsbury, Earl of, *The Laws of England*, (London, 1909), vol. 20, p. 337.

296. New York Civil Practice Act, sec. 352.

297. Regan, op. cit., pp. 80-83.

298. *J.A.M.A.*, 163, 8, (Feb. 23, 1957), p. 702.

299. Regan, L., op. cit., p. 35.

300. A. M. A. *"Principles,"* (as above), ch. 2, sec. 3.

APPENDIX

ETHICAL AND RELIGIOUS DIRECTIVES FOR CATHOLIC HEALTH FACILITIES [1]

— Preamble —

Catholic health facilities witness to the saving presence of Christ and His Church in a variety of ways: by testifying to transcendent spiritual beliefs concerning life, suffering, and death; by humble service to humanity and especially to the poor; by medical competence and leadership; and by fidelity to the Church's teachings while ministering to the good of the whole person.

The total good of the patient, which includes his higher spiritual as well as his bodily welfare, is the primary concern of those entrusted with the management of a Catholic health facility. So important is this, in fact, that if an institution could not fulfill its basic mission in this regard, it would have no justification for continuing its existence as a Catholic health faciity. Trutees and administors of Catholic health facilities should understand that this responsibility affects their relationship with every patient, regardless of religion, and is seriously binding in conscience.

A Catholic-sponsored health facility, its board of trustees, and administration face today a serious difficulty as, with community support, the Catholic health facility exists side by side with other medical facilities not committed to the same moral code, or stands alone as the one facility serving the community. However, the health facility identified as Catholic exists today and serves the community in a large part because of the past

1. Issued by the United States Catholic Conference Department of Health Affairs. Copyright 1971, United States Catholic Conference. Reprinted with permission.

dedication and sacrifice of countless individuals whose lives have been inspired by the Gospel and the teachings of the Catholic Church.

And just as it bears responsibility to the past, so does the Catholic health facility carry special responsibility for the present and future. Any facility identified as Catholic assumes with this identification the responsibility to reflect in its policies and practices the moral teachings of the Church, under the guidance of the local bishop. Within the community the Catholic health facility is needed as a courageous witness to the highest ethical and moral principles in its pursuit of excellence.

The Catholic-sponsored health facility and its board of trustees, acting through its chief executive officer, further, carry an overriding responsibility in conscience to prohibit those procedures which are morally and spiritually harmful. The basic norms delineating this moral responsibility are listed in these *Ethical and Religious Directives for Catholic Health Facilities.* It should be understood that patients and those who accept board membership, staff appointment or privileges, or employment in a Catholic health facility will respect and agree to abide by its policies and these *Directives.* Any attempt to use a Catholic health facility for procedures contrary to these norms would indeed compromise the board and administration in its responsibility to seek and protect the total good of its patients, under the guidance of the Church.

These *Directives* prohibit those procedures which, according to present knowledge, are recognized as clearly wrong. The basic moral absolutes which underlie these *Directives* are not subject to change, although particular applications might be modified as scientific investigation and theological development open up new problems or cast new light on old ones.

In addition to consultations among theologians, physicians, and other medical and scientific personnel in local areas, the Committee on Health Affairs of the United States Catholic Conference, with the widest consultation possible, should regularly receive suggestions and recommendations from the field, and should periodically discuss any possible need for an updated revision of these *Directives.*

The moral evaluation of new scientific developments and legitimately debated questions must be finally submitted to the teaching authority of the Church in the person of the local bishop, who has the ultimate responsibility for teaching Catholic doctrine.

Section I: ETHICAL AND RELIGIOUS DIRECTIVES

— General —

Directive

1. The procedures listed in these *Directives* as permissible require the consent at least implied or reasonably presumed, of the patient or his guardians. This condition is to be understood in all cases.

2. No person may be obliged to take part in a medical or surgical procedure which he judges in conscience to be immoral; nor may a health facility or any of its staff be obliged to provide a medical or surgical procedure which violates their conscience or these *Directives*.

3. Every patient, regardless of the extent of his physical or psychic disability, has a right to be treated with a respect consonant with his dignity as a person.

4. Man has the right and the duty to protect the integrity of his body together with all of its bodily functions.

5. Any procedure potentially harmful to the patient is morally justified only insofar as it is designed to produce a proportionate good.

6. Ordinarily the proportionate good that justifies a medical or surgical procedure should be the total good of the patient himself.

7. Adequate consultation is recommended, not only when there is doubt concerning the morality of some procedure, but also with regard to all procedures involving serious consequences, even though such procedures are listed here as permissible. The health facility has the right to insist on such consultations.

8. Everyone has the right and the duty to prepare for the

solemn moment of death. Unless it is clear, therefore, that a dying patient is already well-prepared for death as regards both spiritual and temporal affairs, it is the physician's duty to inform him of his critical condition or to have some other responsible person impart this information.

9. The obligation of professional secrecy must be carefully fulfilled not only as regards the information on the patient's charts and records but also as regards confidential matters learned in the exercise of professional duties. Moreover, the charts and records must be duly safeguarded against inspection by those who have no right to see them.

10. The directly intended termination of any patient's life, even at his own request, is always morally wrong.

11. From the moment of conception, life must be guarded with the greatest care. Any deliberate medical procedure, the *purpose* of which is to deprive a fetus or an embryo of its life, is immoral.

12. Abortion, that is, the directly intended termination of pregnancy before viability, is never permitted nor is the directly intended destruction of a viable fetus. Every procedure whose sole immediate effect is the termination of pregnancy before viability is an abortion, which, in its moral context, includes the interval between conception and implantation of the embryo. [Catholic Hospitals are not to provide abortion services based upon the principle of material cooperation. (NCCB/USCC, Nov. 1973]

13. Operations, treatments, and medications, which do not directly intend termination of pregnancy but which have as their purpose the cure of a proportionately serious pathological condition of the mother, are permitted when they cannot be safely postponed until the fetus is viable, even though they may or will result in the death of the fetus. If the fetus is not certainly dead, it should be baptized.

14. Regarding the treatment of hemorrhage during pregnancy and before the fetus is viable: Procedures that are designed to empty the uterus of a living fetus still effectively attached

to the mother are not permitted; procedures designed to stop hemmorhage (as distinguished from those designed precisely to expel the living and attached fetus) are permitted insofar as necessary, even if fetal death is inevitably a side effect.

15. Cesarean section for the removal of a viable fetus is permitted, even with risk to the life of the mother, when necessary for successful delivery. It is likewise permitted, even with risk to the child, when necessary for the safety of the mother.

16. In extrauterine pregnancy the dangerously affected part of the mother (e.g., crevix, ovary, or fallopian tube) may be removed, even though fetal death is foreseen, provided that:

    (a) the affected part is presumed already to be so damaged and dangerously affected as to warrant its removal, and that

    (b) the operation is not just a separation of the embryo or fetus from its site within the part (which would be a direct abortion from a uterine appendage), and that

    (c) the operation cannot be postponed without notably increasing the danger to the mother.

17. Hysterectomy, in the presence of pregnancy and even before viability, is permitted when directed to the removal of a dangerous pathological condition of the uterus of such serious nature that the operation cannot be safely postponed until the fetus is viable.

II. Procedures Involving Reproductive Organs and Functions

18. Sterilization, whether permanent or temporary, for men or for women, may not be used as a means of contraception.

19. Similarly excluded is every action which, either in anticipation of the conjugal act, or in its accomplishment, or in the development of its natural consequences, proposes, whether as an end or as a means, to render procreation impossible.

20. Procedures that induce sterility, whether permanent or temporary, are permitted when:

    (a) they are immediately directed to the cure, diminution, of prevention of a serious pathological condition and are not directly contraceptive (that is, contraception is not the purpose); and

    (b) a simpler treatment is not reasonably available. Hence, for example, oophorectomy or irradiation of the ovaries may be allowed in treating carcinoma of the breast and metastasis therefrom; and orchidectomy is permitted in the treatment of carcinoma of the prostate.

21. Because the ultimate personal expression of conjugal love in the marital act is viewed as the only fitting context for the human sharing of the divine act of creation, donor insemination and insemination that is totally artificial are morally objectionable. However, help may be given to a normally performed conjugal act to attain its purpose. The use of the sex faculty outside the legitimate use by married partners is never permitted even for medical or other laudable purpose, e.g., masturbation as a means of obtaining seminal specimens.

22. Hysterectomy is permitted when it is sincerely judged to be a necessary means of removing some serious uterine pathological condition. In these cases, the pathological condition of each patient must be considered individually and care must be taken that a hysterectomy is not performed merely as a contraceptive measure, or as a routine procedure after any definite number of Cesarean sections.

23. For a proportionate reason, labor may be induced after the fetus is viable.

24. In all cases in which the presence of pregnancy would render some procedure illicit (e.g., curettage), the physician must make use of such pregnancy tests and consultation as may be needed in order to be reasonably certain that the patient is not pregnant. It is to be noted that curettage

of the endometrium after rape to prevent implantation of a possible embryo is morally equivalent to abortion.

25. Radiation therapy of the mother's reproductive organs is permitted during pregnancy only when necessary to suppress a dangerous pathological condition.

III. Other Procedures

26. Therapeutic procedures which are likely to be dangerous are morally justifiable for proportionate reasons.

27. Experimentation on patients without due consent is morally objectionable, and even the moral right of the patient to consent is limited by his duties of stewardship.

28. Euthanasia ("mercy killing") in all its forms is forbidden. The failure to supply the ordinary means of preserving life is equivalent to euthanasia. However, neither the physician nor the patient is obliged to use extraordinary means.

29. It is not euthanasia to give a dying person sedatives and analgesics for the alleviation of pain, when such a measure is judged necessary, even though they may deprive the patient of the use of reason, or shorten his life.

30. The transplantation of organs from living donors is morally permissible when the anticipated benefit to the recipient is proportionate to the harm done to the donor, provided that the loss of such organ(s) does not deprive the donor of life itself nor of the functional integrity of his body.

31. Post-mortem examinations must not be begun until death is morally certain. Vital organs, that is, organs necessary to sustain life, may not be removed until death has taken place. The determination of the time of death must be made in accordance with responsible and commonly accepted scientific criteria. In accordance with current medical practice, to prevent any conflict of interest, the dying patient's doctor or doctors should ordinarily be distinct from the transplant team.

32. Ghost surgery, which implies the calculated deception of the patient as to the identity of the operating surgeon, is morally objectionable.

33. Unnecessary procedures, whether diagnostic or therapeutic, are morally objectionable. A procedure is unnecessary when no proportionate reason justifies it. *A fortiori,* any procedure that is contra-indicated by sound medical standards is unnecessary.

Section II: THE RELIGIOUS CARE OF PATIENTS

34. The administration should be certain that patients in a health facility receive appropriate spiritual care.

35. Except in cases of emergency (i.e., danger of death), all requests for baptism made by adults or for infants should be referred to the chaplain of the health facility.

36. If a priest is not available, anyone having the use of reason and proper intention can baptize. The ordinary method of conferring emergency baptism is as follows: the person baptizing pours water on the head in such a way that it will flow on the skin, and, while the water is being poured, must pronounce these words audibly: *I baptize you in the name of the Father, and of the Son, and of the Holy Spirit.* The same person who pours the water must pronounce the words.

37. When emergency baptism is conferred, the chaplain should be notified.

38. It is the mind of the Church that the sick should have the widest possible liberty to receive the sacraments frequently. The generous cooperation of the entire staff and personnel is requested for this purpose.

39. While providing the sick abundant opportunity to receive Holy Communion, there should be no interference with the freedom of the faithful to communicate or not to communicate.

40. In wards and semi-private rooms, every effort should be made to provide sufficient privacy for confession.

41. When possible, one who is seriously ill should be given the opportunity to receive the Sacraments of the Sick, while in full possession of his rational faculties. The chaplain must, therefore, be notified as soon as an illness is diagnosed as being so serious that some probability of death is recognized.

42. Personnel of a Catholic health facility should make every effort to satisfy the spiritual needs and desires of non-Catholics. Therefore, in hospitals and similar institutions conducted by Catholics, the authorities in charge should, with the consent of the patient, promptly advise ministers of other communions of the presence of their communicants and afford them every facility for visiting the sick and giving them spiritual and sacramental ministrations.

43. If there is a reasonable cause present for not burying a fetus or member of the human body, these may be cremated in a manner consonant with the dignity of the deceased human body.

Sources:

Final paragraph of Preamble: Vatican II *Constitution on the Church,* #27

Directive

  3 *Pacem in Terris,* n. 11
11 Vatican II: *The Church in the Modern World,* n. 51
18 *Humanae Vitae,* n. 14
19 *Humanae Vitae,* n. 14
20 *Humanae Vitae,* n. 15
28 Vatican II: *The Church in the Modern World,* n. 27
42 Directory for the Application of the Decisions of the Second Ecumenical Council of the Vatican Concerning Ecumenical Matters, n. 63
43 *Canon Law Digest,* Vol. 6, p. 669

INDEX

on mission of the church, 9
on natural law, 12
and non-infallible teaching, 10-11
Vivisection, 102-104
Voluntariety, 22
obstacles to, 25-27
Voluntary act
moral determinants of, 22-25
nature of, 22-23
Withdrawal method
as contraceptive, 244
World Health Organization
code of, 3